BREATHE

ESSAYS FROM A RECOVERING PARAMEDIC

BY

MARIANNE PAIVA

D0973481

Memoir
BOOKS
Chico, CA

BREATHE: ESSAYS FROM A RECOVERING
PARAMEDIC

Copyright © 2011 by Marianne Paiva
Cover art by Kyle Wade

ISBN: 978-0-9793387-9-3
Library of Congress Control Number 2011931066

Printed in the United States of America
First Edition

Memoir Books
An Imprint of Heidelberg Graphics
2 Stansbury Court
Chico, California 95928

Contents

DEDICATION

*For my children
Nicholas,
Evelyn Elizabeth,
and Cristopher*

ACKNOWLEDGEMENTS

As with any work of this type, there are many people other than the one doing the work who deserve credit for the success.

Dr. Tony Waters, who has served tirelessly for over a decade as my mentor and most honest critic; it would do any writer well to have someone like Tony in his or her corner. Because of Tony, I am no longer afraid of the red pen. Claire Braz-Valentine and the wonderful group of writers who guided me and listened to these stories first; they forced me to write, even when it often felt too overwhelming.

I am blessed with a team of family and friends who have been at my side every step; I am lucky to be Tony and Nora's daughter, Kerri and Kelly's sister, Matt's wife, and Nicholas, Evelyn, and Cristopher's mom.

There have also been a handful of friends who helped with the very early editing and review of this book, all who said, "keep writing." Thanks to Lisa, Debbie, Sheri, Vianey, Elisa, and one of my favorite teachers ever, Dan Humphers (Go Giants!), for your kind words.

I had many paramedic and EMT partners over the four years I was on the ambulance, too many to count. Some I worked with for only a day or two; others, like Martin and Jon, were coworkers from the first day to the last. Although I mention a few of my partners in this book—David, Martin, Dean—it is usually in passing and briefly. Where I felt it was important, I took mental snapshots of my partners and included them here and there. I have not asked my former partners if I could write about them and do not believe that I can speak for them. And while they are all unique in their own ways, there are several calls in these pages where I cannot remember who my partner was. Even when I can recall, I've still tried to keep information about my fellow paramedics and EMTs out of the story. It's not my place to tell their stories.

I spent four amazing years learning from and working with many emergency medical technicians, paramedics, nurses, doctors, pilots, law enforcement officers, and firefighters who deserve credit for their work in these pages. Their work is not unnoticed or unappreciated. But these stories are about the patient, always first, and then, about my interaction with them. My partners and I are not the most important thing here.

A few colleagues I must mention specifically, though, are those who have passed away: Ron "Jonesy" Jones, Chuck Jerpe, Lisa Gonzalez, Michael Sanchez, and Jeff Davis; my sincere thanks for the lessons you bestowed on your journey. Each of you was lost too soon but your life's work lives on in your patients, the colleagues you mentored, and the hundreds of emergency workers who got to ride along with you even for a day. It was my privilege to know you.

AUTHOR'S NOTE

EXCEPT WHERE NOTED, the following events occurred between June 1, 1993, and April 1, 1997. I have attempted to recreate each event to the most accurate account my memory will allow. I have taken creative license with certain details of the stories, such as color of clothing and types of vehicles, when my memory failed to accurately recall specifics. I have attempted to stay as close to the truth as possible throughout.

To protect the identity of my patients and colleagues, I have changed names where appropriate.

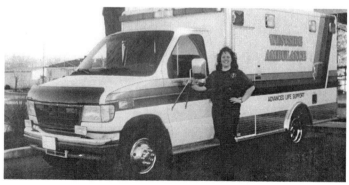

Marianne Paiva, Orland, California, 1995

RECOVERING PARAMEDIC

EACH DREAM IS the same; it begins deep in the night when sleep is heaviest. But instead of being in my bed, I feel the grip of a warm steering wheel in my hands and to my right, my former partner, Martin, sits in the passenger seat of the ambulance. The radio squawks its incessant warning over and over: structure fire out in one of the barns on a backcounty road. We have been called to stand by while the volunteer fire department attempts to quell the flames of a thousand bales of dry alfalfa sending pillars of smoke high into the valley sky. Martin speaks into the radio and I drive, no lights, no sirens, toward the smoke a few miles away. He is confident and sure of himself, his actions. Somewhere in the back of my mind, the Sleeping Marianne tells the Dream Marianne that it's time to wake up, that Sleeping Marianne shouldn't be dreaming about being back on the ambulance, but Dream Marianne ignores her counterpart and continues on. *You gave up your license,* Sleeping Marianne tells Dream Marianne.

I have to be here, Dream Marianne responds.

Dream Marianne glances toward Martin; a smile warms her face. In my dream, Martin meets my eyes, returns my smile, nods his head in acknowledgment, and turns toward the path ahead. The setting sun fills the cab of the ambulance, and as the glow of the late afternoon light warms my face, I know I am home. I am home.

THE BOY

THE BOY LAY on the rough pavement, his eyes closed, his back pressed against the cold, unrelenting surface. His tiny body, perhaps four, four and a half feet long and sixty or seventy pounds, stretched to its full length and then some, the broken bones throughout his skeleton pressing their way through the layers of muscle and skin surrounding them. The splintered mid-shaft of a femur protruded from the middle of one narrow thigh.

Ribs, broken in uncountable numbers, struggled to hold the integrity of the chest, failing miserably from the pressure of gravity. His lungs struggled to grasp the smallest amount of air, anything to feed the dying cells and tissue. He could have been only sleeping, had it not been for the blood flowing profusely from his head. The implement of his demise, the American sedan with the crumpled grill, rested less than twenty feet away.

Standing over the boy, assessing the injuries, not one by one, but through level of significance, the paramedic's mind races and catalogs the necessary treatment. What needs to be done first, second, third? The helicopter is racing through the valley sky toward us; firefighters are stopping traffic, and police have detained the driver and are holding back both do-gooders and onlookers. The scene was set and suddenly, this dying boy with no chance at life, whose life was shattered the moment he stepped into the intersection on his way to school on a brisk October morning, has taken center stage, and we are his supporting cast.

He needs to be intubated (the procedure of inserting a plastic tube into the trachea to assist respiration), an intravenous line needs to be inserted. We need to begin CPR as soon as his heart stops working. And the bleeding, we need to stop the bleeding from his head. It is strange that there is very little blood except from the head. Even the femur—sticking up so defiantly—has bled minimally, compared to the head. The blood, so bright and clean, has formed a red halo around his short blond hair and the warmth of it steams against the cold blacktop. All the other injuries he may have lived through but that wound on the back of his head, where I am sure the brunt of the impact focused, will, in a matter of minutes, kill him.

I open his eyes to gauge the depth of his brain injury, staring at the pupils long enough to see that he is already dead. The pupils of the eye reflect the anatomical structure of the brain; the pupils have fixed and dilated meaning the hemispheres of his brain have ruptured. Both hemispheres of the brain have been compromised and with that, all higher brain function will inevitably, rapidly, cease. His heart will beat and the lungs will try to breathe, but the brain has already died and there is nothing I, or any other human, can do to save this child.

It is my job, though. It is my responsibility to perform the necessary functions, intubate, defibrillate, medicate. The voice inside my head, the one that says, "Do your job," tells me to assemble my equipment, kneel before this child, breathe for him, compress the heart muscle if need be, be the barrier, if only for a little while, between life and death.

The rest of my consciousness knows that measures we take will only violate the tiny body with tubes and medicine and procedures, trying to revive or prolong the life that is already gone.

SMALL TOWN GIRL

I LEFT THE ambulance in 1997 and I began writing this in the summer of 2006, nine years after my last call. This book began as a request from a friend who was thinking about becoming an emergency medical technician. "Marianne," my friend Michael wrote in an e-mail, "what's it really like to be an EMT? Are there any books you can recommend that would give me some insight?" I responded that although there were several fine books written by EMTs or paramedics about working on an emergency ambulance, there wasn't one that came close to what my experiences had been. And it doesn't help to say, "It's really stressful, it's gruesome at times, the pay isn't great, and the hours are tough," because that could just as easily describe an exterminator's day as a paramedic's. Instead, in that e-mail, I wrote the first draft of "The Toothache," a story included here.

These stories begin in 1993. I had taken a first aid class in the spring of that year and realized that with a small child in the house, I didn't know enough about how to save him in case of an emergency. When the local community college offered a six-week EMT course over the summer, I jumped at the chance to enroll. I spent half of June and most of July in a classroom and hospital learning how to perform patient examinations and apply splints and bandages and slings to broken and bloody extremities. As a class, we spent several afternoons extricating our classmates from a beat-up 1970s American sedan. I still remember the first time I heard the "thump, thump, thump" of the blood rushing under the gauge on the blood pressure cuff. And I remember the day I fainted in the hallway of the emergency department after I watched a doctor stitch up a three- or four-year-old boy's forehead. As I lay on a gurney, a janitor walked by and said, "You'll never make it" and continued sweeping the shiny linoleum floor. At the end of the six weeks, I passed an exam and a month later, the state sent my EMT certificate. I was, according to the State of California, qualified and certified to respond to medical emergencies and care for ill and injured patients.

I landed my first job as an emergency medical technician on an emergency ambulance in November of 1993. Six weeks later, on December 26, I realized that if I was to stay on the ambulance, I needed to know more about medicine.

As an EMT, I was restricted to caring for the few patients who didn't need an IV, medication, cardiac monitoring, or advanced airway control. Almost invariably, I drove the ambulance to the hospital while the medic, licensed to perform advanced emergency medical treatment, cared for the patient. I spent eight months responding to traffic collisions, cardiac arrests, and drug overdoses, watching nearly helplessly as my paramedic partners administered life saving medications and intubated patients in respiratory distress.

I finished the prerequisites for the Mobile Intensive Care Paramedic program—anatomy, psychology, algebra, English—by the summer of 1994. That fall, I enrolled in the Mobile Intensive Care Paramedic course at Butte Community College where I had completed my EMT training, graduating in May of 1995.

On May 31, 1995, I served my first shift as a paramedic in my hometown.

My last call came on the morning of April 1, 1997.

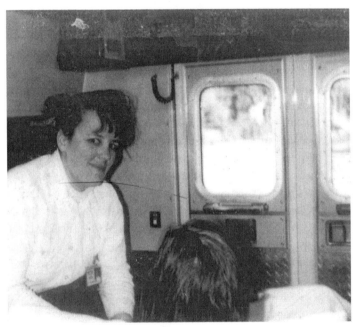

Marianne Paiva tends a patient on their way to the hospital.

ORLAND

My HOMETOWN, ORLAND, in the northern part of Glenn County of the Central Valley of California, and where I spent most of my time on an ambulance, is one of the hundreds of small farm towns that dot the Central Valley along Interstate 5 and Highway 99. From the tops of the Interstate 5 overpasses on the west side of town, Mount

Shasta is visible, its perpetually snowcapped peak outlining the marker for due north.

In the mid-1990s, Orland boasted two stoplights and around 5,000 residents. There was no McDonald's, Walmart, or AM/PM. Only Taco Bell, Burger King, and Subway have managed to appease the city council and today, one of each restaurant sits at the north freeway off-ramp. Orland had, and still has, only one elementary, one middle, one junior high, and one high school. But the town is growing; when I started kindergarten at Mill Street Elementary in 1977, there were only four kindergarten classes. By 1995, there were eleven.

The community raises working class ranchers, mechanics, dental assistants, store clerks, and schoolteachers in Orland. They are the children of farmers and farm workers, small business owners, and the clerks at the local grocery store. Many of our patients' grandparents arrived from the Midwest in the 1930s as seasonal farm workers and stayed. Others were the children of Mexican farm workers who had settled there in the 1970s after following the migrant farm work up and down the Pacific Coast. By the 1990s, a division between the two groups had emerged. In the 2000 presidential election, 65 percent of the voters favored Republican George W. Bush over Democrat Al Gore.

My sisters and I grew up ten miles south of Orland, out in the county on an eighty-acre almond ranch. We weren't necessarily farm kids; my sisters were cheerleaders and we all played on the tennis or softball teams after school. We weren't city kids either; my sisters also had farm animals they raised and sold at the county fair. We lived ten miles from the nearest grocery store and, every day, we rode the bus over an hour each way to attend school. We ran rodeo on the weekends and followed my oldest sister Kerri to the California State Rodeo Finals in 1982, where she placed thirteenth in the state in pole bending.

We listened to Barbara Mandrell, Waylon Jennings, Dolly Parton, and George Jones on the radio. Each summer, our closest neighbors held dances in an oversized red wooden barn a quarter mile down the road. We stood on our front lawn and watched the lights of the party between the slats of the barn and danced to the music that radiated through the hot July evenings. We picked baby ears of corn from the tall green stalks in the field behind our house and learned to swim in the irrigation ditches that ran through the orchards. When I was very young, Dad would bring sick or abandoned sheep, calves, and pigs home. For weeks, the animals would live in our back porch and we hand-fed them until they were big enough to get by on their own.

We started driving tractor and Dad's pickup by the time we were four or five. "Just keep 'er straight, Marianne, you'll be fine," Dad would say after he propped me up on books and pieces of wood behind the wheel of his hay truck.

"But Daddy, I can't see!" I would wail.

"See that big pole right there," he would point to a tall telephone pole.

"Uh huh." I couldn't see the field or hood of the truck in front of me, but the pole jutted high into the sky; I could see that.

"Head toward that pole, both hands on the wheel."

"Okay," I would reply. Dad would put the truck in first gear and shut the door as he stepped into the field filled with yearling calves. My hands vibrated softly on the big steering wheel and together, we made long passes in the field, me driving and Dad opening bales of alfalfa hay, tossing the loose leaves to the calves.

We worked in the orchard during harvest and slept out on the front lawn in the summer when it became too hot in the house to sleep. The mosquitoes would hum and bite all night long and in the morning, we would be covered in large, itchy aggravating welts.

We knew the neighbors in Orland, even though they were four miles up the dirt road and another mile down another one. There were four houses on our six-mile long road when I was a kid. The new neighbors built their place on the corner in '83 or '84, making the total five, which hasn't changed in over twenty years. They've moved on; they were there only ten years or so. When I was eleven, my mom and I drove down to their new home and introduced ourselves to the young family. Pam was very pregnant with Kyle while Clint played on the floor as we visited. I babysat the boys until I was sixteen or seventeen; Clint spent time in the military and returned home, but it was Kyle we lost in 2005 in a tragic boating accident.

We waved at the oncoming cars that passed on the mostly deserted back roads that lead to town, just a small flick of the index and middle fingers off the steering wheel, a slight nod of the head in return. Sometimes, the driver was a stranger taking the back roads between Interstate 5 and Highway 99. But mostly, it was one of our neighbors headed to the field or office, or headed home from the grocery store. I once made the teenaged mistake of not waving at a car on our road and at dinner that evening, my mother asked why I hadn't waved at Irma, our closest neighbor since 1966. I had no excuse, but just dropped my head and stared at the tuna casserole with crumbled potato chips on top as it cooled on the plate in front of me.

When my first article appeared in the local newspaper, the *Chico Enterprise Record,* in 2004, my dad's neighbor, Ernie, clipped it from the newsprint and made a special trip to deliver it to my dad. He remembered me from when I was a young girl. Dad had bought the dairy a couple of miles from his own. Dad and I would stop by Ernie's on our way to town, or we'd stop by to pick up hay or feed.

When I got older, I walked by Ernie's house on the way to swim in the creek. I still have the scar on the palm of my hand, clean as the cut of a surgeon's scalpel, from the open end of an irrigation pipe I grazed at the bottom of the creek when I once dove too deep. The narrow, pale line runs from the base of my thumb toward the center of my wrist, not quite reaching the arm.

Orland's the type of town most people believe they would like to raise kids in, although sometime in the last twenty years, it's gotten a little bigger and there are more strangers stopping and staying instead of passing through. With each addition, the town becomes a little less friendly. Even though its still growing and changing, Orland's still my hometown. I no longer live there but every once in a while, I miss the feel of freshly tilled dirt between my toes and the smell of just-cut alfalfa on the wind.

MEDICAL RESOURCES IN GLENN COUNTY

IN THE EARLY to mid-1990s, two ambulance companies served Glenn County. Valley Emergency Medical Services, where I worked from 1993 to 1995, contracted for the southern portion of the county, which includes Willows. They were a for-profit company. Valley EMS employed a mix of paramedics and emergency medical technicians, some with advanced certification in medication administration and cardiac care. One paramedic (or advanced certified EMT) and one EMT-basic staffed one ambulance per twenty-four-hour shift.

For a while, we were housed in an aging strip mall directly across the street from the hospital. "Quarters" included a front office where we could sit to finish our paperwork, a small kitchen, a full bathroom, bedrooms for crewmembers, and a small conference room. When part of the in-patient section of the hospital closed, they moved us to the empty wing where hospital beds had been replaced with regular beds and we showered in cold, industrial bathrooms that didn't have real curtains or doors. We used the nearly abandoned staff break room to microwave TV dinners and popcorn. At night, when my paramedic partner fell asleep or went to the ER to visit the doctors and nurses, I turned out all the lights and slid up and down the over-waxed linoleum floors in my socks, dancing like Tom Cruise in *Risky Business*. It passed the time on those too quiet nights, when I worried about being a twenty-two-year-old woman alone in the nearly empty hospital. I had read too many suspense novels and imagined a murderer lying in wait for my male partner to leave or for me to take a shower in the evenings. There were no locks on the bathroom doors. I would have been easy prey.

The northern part of the county—everything north of County Road 34, which includes Orland and Hamilton City—fell into Westside Ambulance's territory. They are a nonprofit organization, governed by a board of directors, whose sole purpose is to ensure Orland and the surrounding area has advanced ambulance services. They have succeeded, for the most part, in their mission. In the early 1990s, through donations from the community, they built a two-bedroom house with oversized garage to house the crew, small staff, and ambulances. The board was also able to secure funding to equip two state-of-the-art ambulances for our crews. I worked at Westside from 1995 to 1997, at which time we staffed one ambulance each twenty-four-hour shift with two paramedics. We averaged just over two emergency calls a day, although there was a stretch of nearly three days once, that we had no calls at all.

Glenn Medical Center is the only hospital in Glenn County with an emergency room. It was never a large hospital with only ten or twelve beds at its busiest. A generation or two of babies have been born there and countless pairs of tonsils removed, but over the last decade, funding has cut its hours and staffing to a skeletal existence. In the early 1990s, a single doctor and one or two registered nurses staffed the emergency department on each eight-hour shift. Another nurse and nurse's aid usually watched over the two or three patients who occupied the in-patient ward on any given night. When I worked in Glenn County, Drs. Dayan and Sanchez were the two who most frequently ran the department. On slow nights, my partner and I would walk across the street from our run-down strip mall or through the darkened hallways of the nearly abandoned hospital to the emergency department. Dr. Dayan often ordered Chinese food and sodas for the ambulance crew and together, we would sit until the early morning hours watching the grainy reception of the nineteen-inch color television suspended in the corner of the eight-person waiting room of the ER. The receptionist, usually Cathy or Teri, would shake her head at us from behind the long, low white desk that sat just inside the doors of the ER. Cathy finished her college degree at Chico State sitting behind that desk. When the telephone rang for me or when I had forgotten to complete a form, she would yell across the tiny waiting room or down the long hallways, "*Mare-ee-anne!* Girl, what are you thinking?" She made my name three full words. She would hold the paperwork over her red-tinted hair and roll her bright blue eyes as I ran toward the desk and snatched the phone or papers from her hand. She kept me in line and more than once, saved me from myself when I failed to write a report thoroughly.

The hospital was small and over time, had become slightly run down. But the staff worked tirelessly on patients that happened into their lives. I never saw one doctor or nurse hesitate to get his or her hands dirty, even with the less desirable patients. Most of them believed, I think, that the next patient could be their son or daughter, husband, wife, or parent. Glenn Medical Center has since been bought out by a larger hospital and the doctors and most of the nurses I worked with have moved on, but it's still the only hospital and has the only on-call doctor in Glenn County.

Even with its limited resources, most people who needed an ambulance in Willows were transported to Glenn Medical due to lengthy travel time to a bigger hospital. Although Glenn Medical Center in Willows is a few miles closer, the hospital most Orland and Hamilton City patients opted to be transported to was Enloe Hospital in Chico, a city of a hundred thousand people, twenty miles from Orland and where the state university is located. Enloe also served as Westside Ambulance's base station hospital; when I needed permission for certain medications or procedures, I called the Enloe Emergency Department to get the orders. With nearly four hundred beds, Enloe is much larger than neighboring Glenn Medical Center. Enloe is the place where all critical and trauma patients are transported. Multiple doctors and many nurses staff its emergency department twenty-four hours a day.

An air ambulance helicopter is stationed out of Enloe. It travels high over the city until a few hundred feet from the hospital, then drops from the sky suddenly and lands on the roof of the four-story hospital several times a day. The nurse and paramedic on Flightcare transport only the most critical of patients, or those from remote areas.

TELLING STORIES

IN THE EARLIEST days of writing this book, a friend of my husband's asked what I was doing over the summer. I had gotten over the hesitation of saying "I'm writing a book" so I told Brad, "I used to be a paramedic and lately, the stories have been keeping me up at night. I'm writing a book."

Brad laughed knowingly and said, "I used to be a medic, but I don't have any stories I wanna tell." And then, without any prompting, he told a story. A man, Brad said, was dead from a heroin overdose. He was a big guy, this heroin overdose victim, and his wife wouldn't tell the medics how long he had been down. Brad began treating the guy, "who was about seven feet tall and four hundred pounds and looked like he had been dead for several days." Brad had administered several vials of Narcan, an antidote to heroin, when he saw his patient begin to twitch. They restrained the man and administered two more vials, "FIVE vials!" Brad yelled. "Can you imagine?" Most people wake up after one or two, if they are going to wake up at all. "The guy wakes up! Sits straight up on the gurney and yells, *Who fucked with my high?*"

We tell stories, as paramedics, even when we don't want to. Twenty-five years after Brad left the ambulance, he was still telling stories.

I found, after interviewing many paramedics and talking to even more casually, that telling stories is something most paramedics do; maybe it's the nature of the job, maybe storytellers just tend to become paramedics, I don't know. But, when I wrote the first story here, I knew that it would not be my last and I suspect that in twenty years, I'll still be doing it.

What follows is not a comprehensive collection of the experience of my days on the ambulance; in fact, these are just a few among the hundreds of patients I cared for in my four years on the ambulance. But these are the stories, stories like Brad's heroin overdose, that keep me up at night and haunt me when I drive by the cemetery out on Road

P in Orland where some of my patients are buried. They are the stories I must tell. After reading them, I hope you'll understand why. Don't forget to hold on. And don't worry, I'll take care of you.

JEFF

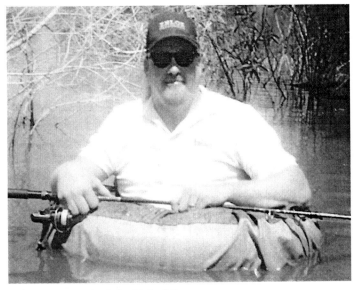

Jeff Davis, paramedic, Enloe Medical Center

IN THE LATE spring of 1995, my days as a student paramedic were numbered and my preceptor, Jeff, had begun to let me work patients without his input. The classroom portion of my training was completed in December of 1994;

followed by a six-week stint at various hospitals in the area.

I learned how to deliver babies during the week I spent in the obstetrics ward at Feather River Hospital and twice, cut the umbilical cord that connected mom and baby. I listened to countless pairs of ragged, wheezing lungs for two weeks in the Intensive Care Unit at Enloe Hospital while on another floor, a young mother who had been stabbed in the back of the neck by her husband was removed from life support. The murderer refused to donate her organs, despite the pleas of her grieving mother. He said, it was rumored, that he didn't want any part of her to live. He was her husband. Legally, the decision was his.

I was given an anatomy lesson in the Emergency Department by a physician suturing a gunshot wound that had penetrated a young man's upper arm and came clean through the other side. "See this," the doctor said as I watched him work, "this is the best kind of gunshot wound; it went in, and came right back out. Didn't even hit any major vessels." He inspected the wound curiously, lifted a flap of skin on the lower bullet hole, laced his smallest finger into the opening, and, a second later, the tip of his glove peeked through the second hole. His finger was nearly covered by the cavity the bullet had made in the victim's arm. I wanted to wince at the unnatural intrusion into the patient's body, but held my face neutral and my body at ease.

I completed my hospital rotations in February. In March, I joined Jeff's ambulance. I would spend a total of twenty shifts, 480 hours, two full months with my preceptor until the State of California and Jeff himself deemed me fit to run my own ambulance. Until then, he was at my side and I ran calls under his experienced eyes. I followed Jeff diligently, watching as he entered chaotic scenes, soothing patients with his oversized confidence and easy silence.

He stood well over six feet tall, towering over most of his patients and all of his colleagues. With a thick goatee, wide shoulders, and light strawberry blond hair, he reminded me of Major League Baseball player Mark McGwire. With sunglasses on, the two could have been twins. Jeff even tried out for the Major's the year the league went on strike and Jeff was still young enough and strong enough to have a shot at the big time.

Jeff was the first choice of a partner for many paramedics and emergency medical technicians, despite his laidback attitude that irritated management. Although he had been in the field ten plus years by the time I joined his crew, he repeatedly refused the supervising paramedic position offered to him and the extra pay that came with it. He had begun his career on the ambulance as a fluke. A flier posted on a bulletin board at the local community college advertising a new paramedic-training course caught his attention when he was just out of high school. He was just a kid when he became a medic, but by the time I worked with him, he was one of the most seasoned in the county. He bypassed the politics and state regulations that came with being a charge medic even though the pay was a little better. Hospital management hounded him every few months to take the increased responsibility, but Jeff always declined. Jeff showed up for work, did his job well, and went home. There was no bullshit to Jeff and he didn't hesitate letting people know exactly where they stood with him, even management when he disagreed with their decisions. Maybe that's why every medic I knew wanted to be partnered with Jeff: good or bad, he spoke the truth. He was honest, and people trusted and appreciated that in him. Plus, he was a damn good medic.

I had known Jeff for nearly four years when he became my preceptor in early spring 1995. I had been nanny to his two small children since 1991. While Jeff worked as a paramedic, his wife Donna worked at the local hospital as a respiratory therapist. They performed long hours. By the time their second child, Haley, was born in March '91, I sat two or three days a week with Tyler, Haley, and my own son Nicholas, usually from before the sun came up to after it set. I was there when Tyler and Haley woke in the morning and read bedtime stories to all three children cuddled together under blankets in the living room.

The boys were born within fourteen months of each other. They learned to walk by copying each other, swam together on hot summer days, and were with me so much that by the time they were two and three years old, I felt like a part of their family. I watched Jeff and Donna go off to their respective jobs each day. Often I would stay over so Jeff could sleep off his twenty-four-hour shift without being disturbed by the kids.

There was something about Jeff and the work he did that intrigued me. Several times I knew he had been on a tough call at work but he wouldn't say a word about it when he came home. He never looked differently, extra stressed, or more tired than usual. Each day was the same: He walked in the door, hugged the kids, unloaded his overnight bag in front of the washing machine in the garage, and I caught him up on the events of the day. "We went to the park, and grocery shopping. Haley took a long nap. We had fish sticks, mac and cheese, and applesauce for dinner," I recounted dutifully.

We would sit at the kitchen table for a few minutes and he would laugh while Haley wiggled herself onto her daddy's lap, and he would tell me it sounded like a good day. As we talked about swinging in the park and the long walk the kids and I took, I watched his face for a hint of the secrets I knew he must carry from the ambulance shift.

In the summer of 1993, when I told him I wanted to take a basic emergency medical technician class, he didn't discourage me. When I joined his ambulance crew two years later for the final portion of my advanced training before I earned my paramedic license, he was my strongest ally. But before he would let me go out on my own, he taught me the most important lessons of my career, and in the process he shared the secrets of the ambulance and the lives of the people he called his patients.

We worked easily together, Jeff and I. Ambulance crews need to trust each other implicitly to run smoothly; I trusted Jeff with my life and even though I had not earned it, I felt, from my first day on his ambulance, that he trusted me also. I learned quickly to listen, watch, and learn from the mistakes and example of others. I paid attention when Jeff criticized another medic as we washed the ambulance on a cool April morning behind quarters. Greg had made an error in a common medication dosage, we learned, as he told us about a bad call he had just returned from. Jeff watched Greg as he walked away from us a few minutes later. He shook his head and twisted a cloth in his large hands, "Greg's been a medic for five years and still doesn't know the correct concentration of epinephrine for anaphylaxsis. He shouldn't be a medic." Jeff gave him one last reproachful glance, turned back to our overwaxed, shiny white and blue striped ambulance, and wiped the last few drops of water from the block letters stenciled on the outside of the large patient compartment.

Jeff made it okay to say, "I don't know how to do that, can you show me?" And he would. From Jeff, I learned how to intubate a real patient, not a manikin like we had practiced in school. I learned how to listen to the rush of blood through a blood pressure cuff and *really* understand what the sounds said about the patient's heart. But what he taught me wasn't entirely technical; during my two months on his watch, I also learned how to read a scene and came to understand the difference between a drug seeker and someone in real pain. I learned patience from Jeff and how to stand taller and stronger when police or firefighters challenged my authority on a scene. Jeff ran calls on intuition, and I learned to listen to my own gut, especially when it whispered, *"something's not right here."*

When I earned my license, it was Jeff I called after the first day on the job, crying uncontrollably at the experience. The charge medic, Dwayne Peters, had grilled me all day on proper procedure, medication dosages, hypothetical call scenarios, and finally had told me, in no uncertain terms, that "I would be sharing" his bed if I wanted to work there. Instead, I lay on the couch in the common area of crew quarters, fully dressed, boots and all, the entire night. He would not force me to leave, but I was terrified that he would force himself on me in my sleep, so I stayed awake and prayed for the morning light to shine through the windows. As I cried into the telephone to Jeff the next morning, I told him that I didn't know if I could make it, if I was good enough or strong enough for the job.

"Marianne," Jeff chastised, "I wouldn't have let you off my ambulance if you weren't good enough."

Although I slept uneasily in quarters for the next two years in fear that Peters, who had threatened me, would find me and take retribution for losing his job, I never again doubted my worth as a medic. Jeff had faith in me and that was enough. Every once in a while, though, he taught me a lesson the hard way.

NARCAN

THE CALL CAME on the seventh day of the safety net when I was working with Jeff.

My seventh duty shift on Jeff's ambulance began at 7:00 a.m. on a bright March day. We washed and stocked the ambulance, found breakfast, and made our way to quarters, where Jeff turned on the old nineteen-inch TV in the living room. The O.J. Simpson trial loomed over the nation and we spent much of our down time transfixed with testimony of the grizzly murders. Jeff tuned the television to one of the cable channels that televised Marcia Clark and Johnny Cochran as they fought over the ex-football star's future. I stretched out on the narrow twin bed in one of the bedrooms and sifted through strips of paper stuffed into a small plastic sandwich baggie. I studied each strip of paper and tried to decipher the message the thin squiggly lines told me. *Normal sinus rhythm, ventricular tachycardia, atrial fibrillation, asystole, wait—Jeff would probably call it fine ventricular fibrillation, we could still shock vfib; asystole or flatlined is unshockable.* I worked through the twenty or so cardiac monitor strips with care; Jeff would test me on the entire bag before the day was over. He would ask what each cardiac rhythm was and then how to treat it:

normal sinus doesn't require treatment, ventricular tachy-cardia calls for Lidocaine to calm the heart down, atrial fibrillation calls for Cardizem, ventricular fibrillation calls for epinephrine, atropine, and defibrillation to jump start the dying heart. The trick is, even though most of the car-diac rhythms look similar, there are tiny differences that can confuse an inexperienced or careless medic. If you give the wrong medication because you aren't paying attention to the small details, the patient could die. Worse, ignore a potentially fatal cardiac rhythm and do nothing for a sal-vageable heart, and you've essentially killed someone.

The call came in the early afternoon, just after lunch and before a quick afternoon nap I had been looking forward to. Jeff dozed on the old couch in the living room but some-how was still ready to go by the time the radio had finished its incessant chirping and the dispatcher had given us the address we would respond to. It was a possible overdose on the south side, not the best part of town, but not the worst. Still, an overdose was not unexpected in the neighborhood. As we drove to the address, I rechecked the protocol for the most likely culprit of the overdose, which was morphine or something similar. We would do nothing if the over-dose was caused by a caustic substance such as rat poison, which I had seen a few times, and we would work the scene as a cardiac arrest if the overdose was cocaine or metham-phetamine induced. Most likely, though, the patient was dead if it was coke or meth; the heart just can't handle the stress of white, sticky powder for too long. But the report from the scene was that the patient was still breathing, al-beit low and slow, was cyanotic or blue at the lips, and was unresponsive. He was a thirty-three-year-old cancer patient with a prescription of liquid morphine that had just been filled, so as I broke open my med kit, I searched the clear glass vials for my weapon of choice: Narcan.

Morphine is an interesting drug. Morphine and its derivatives are one of the most addictive substances available in our medicine cabinets today. It hooks teens who snoop through Mom or Dad's medicine cabinet for interesting looking pills and derails mothers from caring for their children. Oxycontin, a morphine based pill that some doctors are happy to distribute to almost anyone with back pain, sell for twenty or thirty dollars a pill on the street. People beg, borrow, and steal for a taste of Oxy. In small doses, morphine provides great and instant relief from pain. It is one of the first line drugs for angina and dangerously high blood pressure because, within minutes of intravenous administration, it dilates the vessels throughout the body, opening the arteries, veins, and capillaries, allowing blood to flow unobstructed by clots or restrictions in the vessels. Give a dose of nitroglycerin, a few milligrams of morphine, and some oxygen to a patient in the beginning stages of a heart attack and the patient can often avoid any long-term damage to the heart muscle. The most interesting thing about morphine, though, is the ease in which its effects can be reversed with one vial full of Narcan.

But my patient was not a drug addict, in acute pain, nor dying from heart disease. He was, until three weeks before the call on that spring day, a healthy thirty-three-year-old man planning his wedding to his longtime sweetheart, working and living his life finally free of the brain cancer that had been in remission for over a year.

It was a low-slung house in a working-class neighborhood; an old tract home in a neighborhood that, in a few years, would see a resurrection due to an influx of transplants from the Bay Area and Los Angeles trying to find inexpensive housing and retirement in Chico, a still idyllic town of just under 100,000 people. They would bring with them their money and newer cars, buying houses dirt-cheap and selling them a few years later for a tidy profit, moving to bigger houses in better neighborhoods with the proceeds of their good fortune. But in 1995, the house was in mild disrepair and the lawn hadn't been mown in several weeks. A woman in her thirties, pretty and thin but with the telltale signs of recent misery written across her face in artificially early wrinkles and drying tears, met us at the front door. She gestured toward the back of the house and guided us hesitantly through the unnaturally dark rooms. Three older women sat on overstuffed couches in the dimly lit living room, crying softly as we carried our bags of medicine and equipment through the quiet house. They didn't meet my eyes when I glanced toward them and none of them spoke; they only watched as they wiped tears from their sunken cheeks.

The man lay on a mattress in the middle of a room overcrowded with medical supplies and equipment. Cups with straws protruding from their rims sat on a nightstand next to the bed and bottles of prescriptions filled the surface next to the cups, each seeming to vie for its place of importance closest to the dying man. The bed and its sweaty sheets seemed to be creating a hollow around the man's body, sucking him into the mattress and pillows, swallowing him like the earth would swallow him once the cancer had finished its job and killed the last cell in his body. A woman, she was out of place here, motioned us to her side of the bed and said, almost apologetically, "I'm his nurse. He was like this when I got here; I don't know how long he's been down." She gestured toward the little nightstand filled with cups and plastic, orange prescription bottles. I noticed then, one bottle had taken its final stance in front of all the others, closest to the man. The little dark vial, smaller than all the rest, revealed its liquid contents even from the other side of the bed: morphine.

"Is that all he's taken?" I asked the nurse as I dropped my bag to the ground and fell on my knees to the floor beside the man. The nurse shrugged her shoulders and I saw the frustration in her face when I checked to make sure she was still beside me. Then, across the bed, I asked the woman who had greeted us at the front door, "Is that all he's taken?"

She wiped tears from beneath her eyes and nodded. "Yes," she finally sobbed.

Jeff handed an IV setup to me and I quickly wrapped a tourniquet around the man's upper arm. Eric, our EMT, wheeled the gurney into the room while I found a vein to puncture in the man's inner elbow. "Time to go," Jeff motioned to the gurney, and I realized the precious moments I had spent starting and securing the IV were too long.

The young woman stared at the dying man, then bent down to touch the hairline above his wet forehead. "It'll be okay," she whispered through her tears, "I'm coming right behind the ambulance and I'll be with you." She bent to kiss his forehead, then let us lift him from what would have been his death bed to our sterile gurney.

Jeff sat in the jump seat in the patient compartment of the ambulance. We were less than five minutes from the hospital without lights and sirens; at Code Three, we would be at the hospital in half the time. I drew up a vial of Narcan, the antidote to morphine overdose, raised the clear glass so the needle pointed straight toward the ceiling, then pushed the plunger gently, until all the air was pushed out of the vial and a small stream of clear liquid created a fountain effect at the tip of the steel tube. I caught Jeff's eye briefly but he said nothing to me as I prepped the medicine. His arms were crossed loosely over his chest and he smiled at me for the briefest of seconds. I had never used Narcan on a patient before and I took Jeff's silence and smile as approval—I was doing the right thing. Somewhere in the back of my brain I heard a little voice tell me to take it slow, don't push the Narcan fast because it burns the veins, if given too quickly. I stopped myself from plunging the needle in quickly and instead took a deep breath. I counted to five … no time for ten being just one block from the hospital, found the medication port on the IV secured to my patient's arm, and without further hesitation pushed the contents of the vial slowly into the IV.

***

HE LAY ON the thin mattress, shaggy hair sticking in stringy clumps to his forehead. Soft restraints held his wrists to the hospital bed's steel rails, which stood at attention, preventing him from falling off in his drug-induced semi-coma. The fluorescent lights illuminated each pore and crevice his thirty-three years of living had carved into his pale skin and made the mist of sweat on his upper lip glimmer in an unnatural way. The flimsy hospital gown whispered around his thighs whenever he shuffled his legs in unconscious restlessness and every so often, he would swat at an invisible interloper that lit on his face.

I held his hand tightly in mine, his grip strong even in the semi-coma state the emergency room doctor had blissfully ordered through the administration of a morphine drip attached to his inner arm. The needle that delivered the medication dangled partially out of the thin, translucent skin and I watched as each drop of the opiate fell from the bag suspended above the hospital bed, into a small chamber attached to the bag, then down the long, clear tube that connected to the dangling needle. His fiancé had slipped from the room soon after the doctor had him stabilized and I had slipped back in, holding his hand so he wouldn't pull the needle. Every thirty minutes or so, the morphine would wear off or maybe, the Narcan would rear its ugly head again, and the man would wake violently, cursing at me in the slurred speech that was the telltale sign of the brain tumor that worked to steal his life.

Every so often, his arm would start to twitch and the hand I grasped in mine quivered. It hadn't quivered when I had first administered the Narcan in the ambulance, but had instead jerked wildly. His body had echoed the trembling of his limbs and Jeff's large frame held my patient to the gurney for the last minute of the ride in the ambulance. My eyes had felt as wide as saucers as my patient woke grotesquely from the peaceful morphine to the pain and torture of the Narcan and the cancer that worked to eat away at his brain.

His nurse entered the room and pushed a little extra morphine each time he had an episode and when she left, I dropped my head onto my forearms and prayed for forgiveness. I stayed with my patient for several hours in the private emergency room cubicle. The Narcan's ugly grip finally let go of the man's body as late afternoon rolled into the hospital and instead of waking violently when the morphine wore off, my patient opened his eyes and watched me as I sat by his side. I wiped tears from my cheeks and smiled softly at the man.

"Fucking bitch," he slurred through the cancer.

"I-I'm so sorry," I stammered. I let my hand slide from his fingers and reached to press the nurse's call button.

"You shoulda let me die," one side of his mouth drooped and the words tumbled across his tongue awkwardly. He turned his face away.

A room opened for him on the first floor wing of the hospital, where they send patients to die. The wing is filled with the elderly and the gravely ill for whom life saving care is not an option and the phrases "we'll do whatever we can to make you comfortable" and "it's time to call the priest" fill the hallways like helium in a balloon. I found his fiancé during my next shift forty-eight hours later, standing outside my patient's room. I hesitated before I approached her but realized she didn't recognize me; I was just one of a hundred hospital employees. I stopped a few feet in front of her and searched for the right words. Finally, I asked the only thing I wanted to know.

"How is he?" I asked her as she leaned against the sterile hospital wall. She glanced toward me and I watched, as slowly, the light of recognition flickered in her eyes. She lowered her head and studied the pattern of the hallway floor. I stepped back, hoping she would at least acknowledge me.

"He didn't want to die like this, you know," she finally replied. I waited, because there was nothing I could say. She met my eyes and inside, I flinched at what I saw. "He didn't want to die here, in a hospital, with all," she paused and looked up and down the hallway, *"this."*

On the grainy nineteen-inch television, Marcia and Johnny argued over the merits of witnesses and evidence; Jeff watched the scene disinterestedly, his hands working a scrap of toothpick or paperclip. I found a chair in the corner of the sparsely furnished room and planted myself on its aging vinyl seat. I stared at the television and wondered when death had become entertainment. I glanced at Jeff but his eyes did not leave the television. After a few minutes, I made the motions to get up and go to my room, when Jeff finally acknowledged me.

"Where ya been?" he asked, his eyes watching as Johnny Cochran strutted across the small screen. I hesitated before answering; he knew where I had been.

"The hospital," I confirmed. I waited for him to chastise me for checking on my patient but the reprimand never came. Somewhere at the bottom of my soul, I found the nerve to confront Jeff, something I had never done before and that I would never do again. "Why did you let me give him Narcan; you knew what it would do to him."

He watched the television vacantly, fondling the remote control between his large hands. "Will you ever do it again?" he asked without stealing his eyes from the courtroom on the television, "will you ever give Narcan that fast again?"

"No," I replied. I could have waited for more of an explanation, but I knew my time would be futile. Instead, I retreated to my room, pulled the pile of cardiac strips from the small plastic bag, and waited for the next call to come. And wondered, what lesson he would teach me next.

Kenneth

March 1988

The wind blew on the day we buried him. It came from the north, steady and strong enough to sway the tall junipers standing guard as we carried his coffin from the hearse to the narrow spot of earth the groundskeeper had dug for him beneath the maples in the Odd Fellow's Cemetery on Road P just on the outskirts of Orland. His grandmother lies to the south of his grave and to the north, a service road winds its way from the main road past the keeper's shed, on toward the meadow where Miriam and Stacy are buried. On the other side of the shed, Sonny and Isaiah rest only a few plots apart.

He hated the wind, although now I can't remember why, other than it dried everything out and blew dust in our eyes and sometimes, it would push his truck toward the side of the road and scrape the ditch, too close for him. We buried him on my sister Kerri's birthday: March 29, 1988. It was beautiful, sunny, early spring in the valley, except for the wind. The tea length, antique blue dress with the full skirt I wore billowed around my thighs and more than once, I had to push the shiny fabric down to keep it from revealing too much leg. I hadn't eaten since the twenty-fifth, my stomach in knots and my head pounding from lack of sleep and too many hours crying. Someone had pushed a plate of chicken salad into my face the night before, when we had gathered at his mother's home to listen to music and comfort his brother, and although I tried to eat it, I felt guilty a few minutes later and ran to the bathroom, stuck a finger down my throat and vomited the chunks of chicken into the toilet. If he couldn't eat, wouldn't eat—then I would not either.

His name was Kenneth—although his parents called him Scott, his middle name. He hung himself in the garage behind his father's rundown, Spanish cream stuccoed house. He was eighteen years old. He was my boyfriend, the first boy I ever let go all the way. He sang lyrics of his favorite song to me the night he died, the first time I heard Guns 'N' Roses, although in Kenneth's soft quiver, it sounded nothing like Axl Rose.

"You gotta listen to this, Marianne," he said over the phone line. He sang the lyrics of the rock song about heroin and death from the liner notes.

"What's it mean, who's Mr. Brownstone?" I interrupted when he paused to take a breath.

"Its just ... I ... you've got to listen," Kenneth repeated.

"Ok," I gave in, "I'll listen." He sang softly into the phone, his plaintive voice over-pronouncing each word.

"Is that it?" I asked when he had finished.

"Yeah," he said. "It's Guns 'N' Roses."

"What's it mean? I don't understand what he left behind."

Somewhere in the silent, narrow band of the phone line, I felt the disappointment in his voice.

"It doesn't matter, its just a song," he whispered.

His father found him the next afternoon although the

neighbors had seen him through the garage window hanging the previous night. His thin figure, one foot dragging on a wooden chair, looked to them like he was changing a light bulb. "He was always working in the garage," the neighbor said, 'We just thought he was up late.'

But he wasn't just up late and the next day, when he didn't call me before school, my stomach turned; he called me every morning before school, without fail. By noon, when he still hadn't shown up to take me to lunch, my heart raced and my friend Laura offered to drive me to his house to check on him.

"He's fine, Marianne. He probably just slept late," Laura said to me as we drove her mother's heavy sedan away from the high school.

His small white low-rider truck sat in the driveway of his home but when his father answered the front door, hung over from the night before, he said that his son was not home. And no, he didn't know where he was.

We drove back to the high school and waited.

His friend, Mike, found me later that night at Laura's house. I heard his blue El Camino pull into the gravel drive and met him on the front lawn.

"How'd he do it?" I asked Mike.

"Marianne ..." he responded. The tears in his eyes confirmed what I already knew.

"How did he do it?" I demanded. Mike moved to put his arm around my shoulder but I pushed him away.

"Marianne, he's dead," Mike said.

"I know he's dead. How did he do it?"

"I'm so sorry," Mike said.

"I know."

THE DAY AFTER VALENTINE'S DAY

PALE GREEN. CARPET, walls, ceiling.

A couch, beige with large, brocaded 1970s flowers. Blankets and clothes in tall, unruly piles strewn around the room. A man on the floor just inside the front door of the house with the dead lawn; the top of his head visible to those outside. I walked around his head and knelt in front of him; his eyes opened when he sensed me watching him.

Firefighters, volunteers, clamored toward the house, led by the cop who parked just behind my ambulance and Dean, who brought my trauma bag. Unlike a good portion of calls I responded to, I would need it this time.

"The helicopter," I whispered to Dean. "Call the helicopter." I felt Dean stop, uncertain of what to do. "Call the helicopter," I repeated, *"now."* He dropped the bag at the front door and turned back toward the ambulance. The firefighters had stopped too; the man's body and my own blocked the entryway and they had no other place to go. I realized they were trying to find a way in, trying to help.

I kneeled low, leaning into the man, watching his eyes, trying to discern what they were telling me. He lay on his right side, one arm tucked under his body. His left arm raised toward me hesitantly and he pointed to somewhere beyond my back. "Who did this to you?" I asked. He shook his head gently, just a half an inch left, then right. "No one," he seemed to say. His eyes held mine intently and somewhere in them, I could see the apology that he had forgotten to tell someone else.

"Sir, did you do this?" He closed his eyes and tears began to drop onto the pale green shag carpet below. He nodded gently, just once. Yes, he had done this to himself.

A firefighter tried to climb over and behind me.

"Stay back, get out," I barked, realizing that the possible crime scene that surrounded me would be compromised a little more with each new set of boots that entered. The tread would pick up the drying blood that was *everywhere* and would make this virtually impossible to analyze. He stopped abruptly and then retreated, content for the moment to let me work. The cop fumbled with his radio and I felt his disapproval. "I need room," I said, "and in about ten minutes, I'll need a landing zone." The cop glanced at my patient and wondered, I am sure, what the hell I was doing. He couldn't see the injury and in fact, couldn't even see the blood just beyond the door. I hadn't seen it until I had walked all the way through the door either. The cop backed away from the entryway hesitantly; he knew that I was trying to get rid of him and didn't like it much.

I glanced at the firefighters waiting on the lawn. For some reason, I wanted to protect them from this scene. They were just volunteers, after all. They didn't get paid to see things like this. There are certain things that, if you saw it, would make you never volunteer again. I had seen it after the boy; after we had sopped his blood from the crosswalk of a busy street, and not the crosswalk he had been walking in when the sedan struck him. There were a few firefighters who never came back. Somewhere inside of me, I knew that if they saw this, at least a few of them might never be able to respond to a call again. "And I need a backboard, and the gurney. " They fell away one at a time until finally, I had my patient alone.

I spoke as calmly as my head would allow, "Sir, where's the knife? Is it still here?" I envisioned someone sneaking up on me, maybe a wife or distraught family member— they sometimes freaked out when their loved one's were injured, didn't realize I was there to help them, and could be using the knife again, only this time on me. But his arm raised again and pointed to the place behind me he had pointed to before. "Its over there?" he nodded again, slowly, carefully. The knees of my jumpsuit, which I had knelt on while I spoke to him, made a faint sucking sound as I moved slowly away from him. He looked embarrassed at the sound. I had been kneeling in the blood from his wound. "Its okay, don't worry. I'm just gonna get the knife and be right back, okay?" I backed away from him, glancing at the piles of garbage and clothing and blankets. I pointed to each pile, "This one? This one? That one?" and in the process, I surveyed the room. From the kitchen, on the opposite side of the living room, to the edge of the front door and even on the pale green ceiling, smears and sprays of blood coated the entire room. There seemed to be no surface left untouched by the brownish-red stains.

I took each step deliberately, careful not to disrupt any of the pooled blood on the shag. I didn't think I would ever find the knife in the mess until finally, he nodded slightly when I pointed to a pile of blankets. As gently as I could, I lifted a pale blue electric blanket. There, tucked in between the folds, lay a large kitchen knife. It was the type you might use to chop a chicken in two, seven or eight inches long with a three-inch wide blade and I understood fully the depth of the man's conviction.

With gloved hand, I picked up the knife at the tip of its

handle, feeling the weight pull my arm. I handed it to the cop standing at the door, careful not to touch any of the congealed blood that still coated the steel blade.

My patient waited for me in the same spot I had left him. The firefighters and Dean were back, not sure what I wanted, what they were supposed to do. Part of me felt guilty for keeping them from my patient, but the other part of me needed to protect him in his greatest hour of despair. No one's darkest hour should be displayed publicly and I knew that when I would finally let another person into the house, his shame would be complete.

I motioned for Dean to bring in the board, and raised my hand to stop others; *my partner and I could do this, just wait.* As soon as he entered the house, Dean finally saw what the man had done to himself and inwardly gasped, a movement I saw but that was shielded from our patient. There were no more questions and for that, I was thankful.

"Its like a textbook," I whispered to Dean. The man, a Latino in his mid-thirties, tried to speak to me, to catch my eye, but the wound prevented words from escaping. I took his hand and talked to him again. "Sir, this is my partner, Dean, and I'm Marianne. We're gonna help you, okay?" He nodded gently, trying to speak again. "Sir, don't try to speak, please. You have a wound, a cut on your neck, that we need to take care of." Of course, saying it was a cut on his neck was like saying the *Mona Lisa* was a painting.

The cut was from ear to ear, beginning at his right, just under the lobe, and ending at his left, a few inches short of the other. The knife must have been freshly sharpened; it had done its job with clinical effectiveness. The gaping hole spanned at least ten inches in length and opened from the top of his neck to the start of his chest a good six inches or more, the anatomy of his neck displayed like a filleted fish. I wished, for a brief moment, that I had a camera.

Dean slid the backboard behind our patient as I started to prepare my IV and find a vein in his hand. But when I let my hand fall from his, he grasped it desperately and held me tight, his eyes widening in terror. "I'm not leaving," I promised, "I need to work though. We've got to get you to the hospital." He held on for a moment more, then dropped my hand hesitantly.

Dean and I worked in silence while we prepped him for transport; his veins were flat from losing too much blood and the IV failed to start. The blood pressure cuff barely registered a pressure of 56/0, a very bad sign and I wasn't even positive I had heard the 56. His pulse rate had slowed to 40 or so and I wondered how long he had been bleeding. The pooled blood around his body was tacky with time, and when I touched one of the many smears on the wall, it was dry. But he was still conscious, a miracle at this point and so, while we were inwardly frantic, we had to be outwardly soothing, calming. Each time the man took a breath, tiny bubbles appeared on his trachea; that's how we knew he was still alive.

He had missed the carotid arteries by millimeters. I had a full view of their weak pulsing as I examined his esophagus and behind it, the trachea. The esophagus was sliced, along with the veins just in front of the carotids; but they were veins and didn't have as much blood pressure and when they were cut, their walls had contracted onto themselves, saving the man's life.

In paramedic school they never teach you how to treat a patient who has tried to commit suicide by slitting his own throat. They teach you to bandage a stab wound, a sucking chest wound, a slice on the arm. They tell you how to splint a fractured femur and how to help a baby breath again, but they never tell you how to bandage a throat that has been slit from ear to ear. I think somewhere, they assume that the person will be dead and there will be no need for bandages.

As soon as we had him secured on the backboard—in the position that we had found him, on his side but with pillows and bags of saline and tape to secure his head—we began to move him. Two firefighters carried the backboard to the gurney, and the man, seeing that my hands were free again, grabbed at the closest. We loaded him in the ambulance and I climbed in beside him, my hand clutched in his the entire time. Over the radio I heard the approach of the helicopter, readying to land at the open parking lot of the county fairgrounds a few miles away. They wanted an update; the flight nurse and paramedic wanted to know what we would bring them. Dean drove and talked into the radio at the same time. The flight nurse would tell me later that even though we had told him of the wound, they still had no idea what we meant, until they saw it for themselves. To prevent him from fighting treatment, the flight nurse paralyzed him with a medication not in the paramedic's scope of practice, and then intubated him before the helicopter even lifted off.

The patient left the hospital two days later; his wound stitched closed although the scar would last a lifetime. We would find out later, from the neighbor who had called 9-1-1, that the man's wife had left him the day before, Valentine's Day. She had taken the children and gone. It was around noon when the call came, something I would not have remembered except that's when the neighbor had come home for lunch, saw his neighbor's car in the drive, and decided to stop by. The troubled man answered the door with his throat cut.

Every once in a while, I wonder about him. Did his wife return? Did he attempt suicide again and this time, succeed? I wonder about the determination he must have felt, the commitment to die. I wonder.

BOILING WATER

THE FOG IN the Valley settles in deep and low come November, staying sometimes 'til the new year and every once in a while, all the way to the end of March. They call it tule fog, but I always heard tule fog was patchy, hit and miss, not thick and wet and cold like the blankets that cover northern California in winter. It begins late in the evening, just after the sun goes down, patchy near the river and then spreads for the thirty miles on either side of the Sacramento River. Sometimes, it stays into the morning, and once or twice a year, it will stay all day, but mostly, it just comes at night.

At its best, the fog acts as a wispy veil, hanging between the tops of the trees in tiny breaths of moist air. At its worst, it begins at the river and spreads to the foothills east and west. It is on those nights, usually late in the evening before the drunks are on the road and after the five o'clock commute, that late model sedans find themselves wrapped around telephone poles and plunged into fences and ditches.

On this night, there were no accidents, only the woman who couldn't breath. The call came a little after 4:00 a.m. It seems that the worst medicals happen between midnight and 4:00. It was a shortness of breath, ultimately, the most ambiguous of calls. The baby had come in as a shortness of breath, but so did the man who had been stabbed in the chest. With a shortness of breath call, you never knew what you were going to get.

While my partner David and I had slept, the fog had rolled in. The roads were empty at 4:00 a.m. and in town, with the glow of the streetlights burning the fog away, our ambulance glided through the streets with ease. But this call was a little bit out of town, not too far, maybe two or three miles, but far enough that there were no streetlights and the county stopped painting those white lines on the side of the road for guidance on such nights. Instead, the pocked blacktop faded off the edge into oblivion.

At this hour, unless we have been up all night and would rather be sleeping, we run silent. That is, although we are supposed to run the sirens when the emergency lights are working, we will forego the sirens, sneaking through the early morning like burglars. There usually is no reason to run sirens in the hours just before sunrise; it just pisses off the neighbors and honestly, grates on our nerves. And as I would find out years later, there is only so long you can listen to sirens placed strategically over your head before it begins to damage the fine membranes in your ear.

So we run silent through the thickening fog, responding to a "female, short of breath" just a few miles to the west of town. But somewhere in the fog, along one of the back roads, even though I have spent nearly everyday of my life in my tiny town, we lose our bearings and turn left when we should have turned right. We travel slowly, perhaps only fifteen or twenty miles an hour. The blanket of fog hovers just over the strobe of red lights, just above our heads. The windshield wipers slap rhythmically back and forth, side to side, pushing the light mist from our direct vision. It takes a while to realize we are on the wrong road, headed in the wrong direction.

All the roads in the county run alphabetically north to south, numerically east and west. County Road 3 and FF form the intersection at the far northwest corner of the county and in the southeast, County Roads 67 and XX meet just at the county line. The county is split in half just around County Road 34. Our ambulance responds to everything north; another ambulance responds to everything south.

The female with shortness of breath was somewhere around County Road 9 at County Road H, just up over the freeway and a quick right, not more than four minutes from our station. But for some reason, we had taken a left at County Road H, meandering our way south two miles before a large farmhouse appeared to our right. The fog slowed us considerably and nearly ten minutes had passed since the initial 9-1-1 call had come; the dispatcher had already checked on us once, "Westside fifty-three, ETA?"

"Dispatch, Westside fifty-three. Be advised, thick fog in the area is causing delay. ETA five minutes." David replaced the microphone in its metal bracket.

"Copy, will advise caller. Westside, caller is advising us that patient's distress is increasing."

David grabbed the microphone again. "Acknowledged. Advise patient we are in the vicinity."

But as we approached an intersection where several fields met, I eyed the farmhouse on the right. I realized I had been in it before and that if it was the house I knew, we were nowhere in the vicinity of the caller. David turned the steering wheel of the ambulance to turn left. "Stop!" I cried. "Turn right, just for a minute, turn right." He opened his mouth to protest but remembered that I knew the county better than he did; he wrenched the wheel in the opposite direction and we slowly crept toward the old farmhouse. "Shit," I mumbled, "that's Ingrid Paul's house."

"Is that the house?" David asked hopefully. He made a motion to turn into the drive.

"No, that's Ingrid Paul's house." Recollection flickered in the back of my mind. A blond, nine-year old kid smiled widely in my memory as a small flashlight illuminated her pale features. We were hiding under the covers of her bed, Ingrid telling a tale of a man who didn't have a face. I must have let out a small gasp because her grin widened. Even though I didn't want to hear it, I could feel the climax of the story coming. I hated scary stories. But it was a sleepover, and Ingrid Paul was the most popular girl I knew. She could tell me scary stories all night as long as it meant she liked me. And she obviously did, I had been invited to her house for a sleepover.

The only problem was, her house sat in a field on the corner of County Road 20 and County Road H.

A map of the county popped into my head; I closed my eyes and traced tiny squiggly lines north to south: "3, 7, 9, 12, 14, 16, 18, 20." "Jesus, we're over three miles from the call." David's eyes widened in the dim cab of the ambulance.

"Three miles? How?"

We went the wrong way.

"I don't know; just turn around, we gotta go back." I picked up the mike and depressed the button on the side. "Dispatch, Westside 53. Be advised, ETA to County Road 9 is ten minutes." The radio crackled as I shoved it back into its cradle. I buried my face in my hands. "Jesus, Jesus, Jesus."

"Westside 53, confirm, ETA ten minutes? Do you want fire dispatched?" The dispatcher's voice betrayed the alarm in her thoughts and the urgency of the call; obviously she had been talking to the patient and the situation was deteriorating. I glanced at David but he shook his head; he had heard the panic in the dispatcher's voice. He maneuvered the ambulance faster up the county roads even as the fog enveloped us. He flipped on the siren and ran blind. If there were other cars on the road, hopefully they would hear the siren and move; we wouldn't be able to see them through the fog if they didn't.

"Negative, Dispatch. The fog is lifting, we'll be there shortly."

It took nearly twenty-five minutes to reach the woman's house from the time the call came in. Her husband waited outside for us, even though the fog and mist had dropped the temperature into the low forties. "Where have you been?" he demanded.

It was a little house from the 1950s with clapboard siding and wood shingles. With no streetlights, the house lay in near complete darkness, a single window glowing faintly in the night. The husband led us into his home, glancing back every few seconds to ensure we were following. "She's through here," he called to us. "She's real bad now." We stumbled through a dark kitchen, inadvertently banging the airway and trauma bags against the cupboards as we passed. I couldn't see much in the darkness but could hear the low hum of the house as it slept. The refrigerator droned weakly; the kitchen faucet "drip, dripped" as I walked by. As we neared the adjoining living room, a low raspy breath crept toward us. Somewhere near, boiling water bubbled through the darkness.

"She's right in here," he whispered, "she could breath better in here." I did not ask him to explain. As I left the kitchen and found the living room, I understood what he meant.

She was a tiny woman, no more than a hundred pounds

and five feet tall. Her black hair had begun to give way to gray and I guessed she must have been in her early seventies, not much more. She sat in a large rocker, much too big for her dainty frame, outlined in the glow of a small reading lamp—the light I had seen outside. She held a small inhaler to her lips and sucked in deeply, her shoulders rising and falling in concert with each breath.

As I drew closer to her, the sound of boiling water got louder and I wondered briefly why the old man had decided to boil water at this hour. Was he making tea? Coffee? Was he cooking pasta? But I answered my own question as I knelt in front of her. The boiling water was in her lungs.

I understood the quiet of the house, the low lights, her husband's whispered accusations. When death is imminent, there should be peace and comfort. The old man had created that for her.

If there had been no fog, I would have called for the helicopter. The thirty or more minute drive to the hospital would be too long and the helicopter would have made it in ten, the difference between death and life for the woman.

The importance of the lungs is only surpassed by the simplicity of their function. When they are young and fresh, they are one of the three most perfect filters ever created by man or God, second only to the liver and kidneys. Inside the lungs, tiny sacs fill over and over each day, exchanging oxygen, cleaning the lungs endlessly. They take in oxygen from the air and blood from the heart, mixing the two and creating oxygenated blood, sending it back into the heart and body to feed the brain and muscles and cells. But as they age, or when smoke or asbestos or bleach seep in and burn the tiny sacs, the lungs begin to fail and usually there is little to be done that can reverse the process. The end result is often termed chronic obstructive pulmonary disease (COPD), which in reality encompasses a host of ailments that mean that the patient can't breathe. Fluid backs up into the lungs, the little sacs lose their elasticity like an old rubber band forgotten in the back of a junk drawer, and for ten or fifteen years, the sufferer carries a stimulant inhaler and takes daily medication to remove the fluid from the lungs and another to replace the potassium leeched out from the diuretic. It's a cruel cosmic joke played by the drugs the patient relies on to live; take one, and you have to take two more to counterbalance the effects of the first.

The woman hadn't been a smoker, but her husband had been and while he had a persistent cough, it was her lungs that would give out first. They were making their last stand while we were lost in the fog and for a brief second I imagined what terror the couple had endured; he, helpless as he watched his sweetheart die and her, knowing death was near.

She had been through this terror before, although it had never been quite this bad. Every breath she took caused the fragile muscles at her clavicles to retract and the effort it took just to move that much air was taxing her body; she had pushed her body to its end and when she saw us, she closed her eyes and slept. She had had enough.

We have more drugs in our scope to treat respiratory distress than any other ailment. Even heart attacks do not rate as many drugs as respiratory failure. One of the problems with a patient in respiratory distress is that there are so many different causes of that distress: Choking, allergic reaction, drug interaction, asthma, drowning, pulmonary embolism, too many to list. With most respiratory distress patients it's a puzzle, *why can't this patient breathe?* But with the little senior lady, the cause is clear: her lungs are filled with water and she is drowning in her own body. The solution is simple; get the water out of her lungs.

It's always the presumption in prehospital emergency

medicine that we will be able to get the patient to a hospital rapidly; but on this night, that will not happen. It will take at least an hour with the fog and my medications are for quick fixes, just enough to get to the emergency room. Tonight, I will have to stretch my scope of practice to keep the woman alive.

Her husband watches me closely as I open my airway bag and prepare a breathing treatment. My partner opens the trauma bag and extracts an IV set up with a tiny needle; the woman does not need any more fluids, but she does need medications that we will push through the IV. Plus, if she codes, we'll have the line established and will be able to push the epi and atropine immediately to restart her heart. As soon as the IV is secure, David takes a small aerosol can out of the meds bag and hands it to me. I ask the woman to open her mouth and when she does, I shoot a spray of nitro under her tongue.

I need to figure out her medical history, medications she currently uses, if she is suffering any acute pain. I ask the husband a series of questions: How long has she been short of breath? *A little over an hour.* Is she allergic to any medications? *No.* Did she wake up short of breath? *Yes.* Has she taken any medications to help her breathing? *Only the inhaler, but that didn't help much.* I think but don't say, "That inhaler probably saved her life."

"When is she supposed to take her diuretic?" I ask the husband. We need something that will get rid of the water and if she hasn't taken her own medication since the morning before, she can take her own dose of meds, which will be more than I can give her to help her lungs expel the water. I place the breathing treatment nebulizer in the woman's hand but she lets it fall away. I hold the treatment for her and watch as she inhales the bronchodialator that mists up into her face.

"She takes it every morning at 7:00," her husband tells me.

I glance at my watch. Five a.m. is just minutes away; has it been enough time? "Can you get it for me?" I ask. He stares at me, uncertain; I can see the question in his eyes: Does he trust me yet to take care of his wife? Finally, he steps back and disappears down a dark hallway. Our radios don't work in the little house so with my free hand, I pick up the phone on the table beside the recliner. My friend Kathy is working as the charge nurse in the ER and I need her authorization to give the patient her own meds plus mine. I dial the ER direct and wait as the receptionist gets Kathy on the line. David motions to me that he will get the gurney.

"Helllllooooo," Kathy singsongs in my ear. I've seen Kathy take shots of tequila and dance on the table at a local bar; she is one of the best nurses I have ever worked with. "How can I help you Ms. Paiva?"

"Hey Kath, how are you this morning?" I make my greetings, an apology for calling on the landline. My patient's delicate eyes flutter as I speak into the phone.

"I'm good, it's almost time to go home," she replies. "But, how are *you*?" She knows I must be on a call and need her; I never call in the middle of the night without reason.

"Kath, I'm out here on the west side of Orland with a seventy-two-year-old female, severe shortness of breath. History of COPD; woke up around 2:30 with shortness of breath and has since deteriorated significantly."

"Uh huh, uh huh," Kathy encourages. I can hear her pen scribbling furiously in the background.

"She's full of fluid; sounds like she's boiling water in there. Her vitals are fairly stable with a BP of 124 over 90, a pulse rate of 102 and an oxygen saturation of 86. Here's the problem, the fog is too thick to fly the helicopter and it'll take at least an hour to get to you by ground. I've started a breathing treatment, gave her some nitro, and started an IV. I'd like to give her a little morphine to dilate her vessels also, but she's nearly ready for her regular eighty milligram dose of diuretics."

"Uh huh, yeah," Kathy confirms.

"What would you like me to do?" I take a breath and wait for Kathy. The patient's eyes flutter again and she pulls her arm up to swat the nebulizer away. I pull the nebulizer away briefly until she drops her hand, then hold it in front of her face again. This time, she does not bother it.

I can almost see Kathy as she mulls over the information I have given her. *What to do, what to do?* "Ok Marianne, this line is not recorded, just so you know." Yes, I knew that. It was one of the reasons I didn't try very hard to make my radio work: All radio transmissions are recorded. The direct line into the ER is not. "Go ahead and let her take her normal dose of diuretics. How much does she weigh?" I sigh with relief; Kathy has done what I hoped she would do.

"About a hundred pounds."

"Ok, push two milligrams of morphine and five minutes later, give her another nitro. But watch the pressure and her heart rate. If her vitals are still stable, give her two more of morphine. Call me back if she isn't better in ten minutes."

"Thanks Kath, two milligrams of morphine with follow up nitro and two more of morphine if needed. I'll call you when we're on the road."

"See ya girly," Kathy sings, and then the line is dead.

David drives the ambulance slowly across the valley, the fog menacing in its depth. The husband sits in the front passenger seat in the cab; his wife lays on my gurney, a blanket wrapped around her narrow shoulders and her eyes lightly closed. The fluid in her lungs has subsided to a low gurgle and she finally rests, reclined slightly. It takes a little less than an hour for what should have been a thirty-minute trip to the hospital, but the morphine and diuretic and ni-tro worked better than I could have ever hoped and I know my patient will not die tonight. Kathy called twice on the radio, giving me permission to use as much morphine and diuretic I may need and just checking in the last time.

"How ya' doin'?" she asked. And I knew she was more concerned about us driving in the fog and without much sleep than the patient, who I had confirmed was stable, breathing with little effort at that point. "You just take your time," she offered. And as I glanced once again at my rest-ing patient, I knew, that finally, I could.

JACOB

In the evenings and on my days off, I used to pick up CPR and EMT classes to teach at Butte Community College. It didn't pay much, maybe seven or eight dollars an hour for an hour or two, I don't remember. But I didn't do it for the money. Partly, I used the time to brush up on skills that I didn't use often in the field: how to immobilize a fractured collarbone, how to place a splint on a twisted ankle, those things that we rarely were called for. But another part of me liked the students, or rather, the interaction with the students, their eagerness to learn and the fresh perspective they brought to my work. As I taught them how to take blood pressures or listen to the lungs of an asthmatic patient, I would tell them about the fifteen-year-old girl who had been eating peanut butter for years without a problem until one day, she popped open can of extra-crunchy, took one bite, and immediately went into anaphylactic shock. Her father rushed her to the hospital as her lips and fingers and toes turned blue and her chest, bright red. He drove up to the ambulance bay and carried his daughter through the ambulance access doors into the hospital and wouldn't leave her side while the nurses and doctors worked on her.

We would exchange stories about family and friends and dreams, all the while applying neck braces, counting chest compressions and playing "What if?" "What if," one would begin, "you have a patient confined to a wheelchair and they fall out of it? They're already paralyzed; do you immobilize their spine anyway?"

My students were often people I knew from outside of class; people from high school, the clerk at the grocery store, the babysitter my son went to when he was a toddler. I saw them a couple of nights a week in our classroom and the next day at the dry cleaners or the bank; when you live and work in a small town, that's the way it is.

The call came while we were at the gym, lifting weights, on a quiet afternoon. As we sprinted to the ambulance, I stripped off my sweaty t-shirt and running shorts, then slipped into my uniform jumpsuit and steel-toed boots. David drove to the call while I talked to the dispatcher and firefighters who were also called. The call came in as a pedestrian struck by a vehicle just north of Orland on Old Highway 99. As a precaution, I dispatched the helicopter. You never know what you'll find on most calls but a "pedestrian versus auto" on a highway is never a good thing. It took us nearly five minutes to get to the scene; for some reason, cars would just not move out of our way and I cussed loudly at each one that failed to pull over. "Don't they know?" I asked no one in particular. "Do they think that we turn the lights on because they're pretty?"

We drove for another moment in silence, listening to the emergency radio as the helicopter crew was dispatched and then responded. We headed north out of town, passing the used car lot on the left and Gardner's Frosty just a little farther up the road. As we approached the city limits, a large beige arch spanned the road with the single word, "Orland," painted at its apex. Its aspirations were much more than what it turned out to be.

Dispatch told us the "pedestrian versus vehicle" was just north of Stony Creek, so a mile north of the arch, as we crested the bridge that covers the wide waterway, I started scanning the road for our patient.

A line of cars had already formed on the opposite side of the accident scene and those that came from town turned back when they saw the crumpled hood of the late model sedan and several people standing in the middle of the highway. But others had stopped and pulled to the side of the road, cluttering the scene so it made it difficult to assess what exactly had happened just minutes before. The area was sparsely populated, with a cemetery on the right side and a field just beyond, then seven or eight houses in a row dotting the side of the road, most protected and shaded by a canopy of trees that arched over the road.

The battered sedan had pulled to the side of the road at an angle, its grill facing the ditch and its tail end sticking haphazardly into the road. Behind it, a group of people, four or five maybe, were standing in a semicircle, others stood beyond them, out of their own cars but not quite sure what to do. Every few seconds, they glanced furtively to the four in the semicircle and then quickly turned their eyes again.

Our ambulance came to a stop in the middle of the road, a few feet from the battered sedan, but at an angle that shielded the accident scene from our view. I jumped out of the passenger seat and grabbed the trauma bag; David ran around the ambulance and retrieved the airway bag. It was to be his patient; the last patient had been mine. As I ran past the sedan, I glanced at it briefly, taking in the hood, the windshield, the top of the trunk. The dented and crumpled metal of each spot told me more than I wanted to know: Three impacts on the car, one on the pavement. Fuck.

He lay on his back; his body resting where it had come to lie after the car had hit him. Around him, pieces of mail that had fallen from his hands had come to rest like confetti after a New Year's party. He couldn't have been more than fourteen or fifteen years old, his dark hair styled in a long curly mop and his face revealing that he had not yet begun to shave. But he was tall, at least for a boy his age, and thin—probably just going through a growth spurt that boys in mid-teens age are famous for. His eyes were closed and there wasn't much blood; there never seemed to be on calls like this. But his face was too pale and his muscles too slack; something you can't understand until you've seen it yourself. Whenever I see those medical dramas on television treat an unconscious patient who needs to be intubated, I cringe, because I can see the lie in the set of the victim's jaw. The actors, I am sure, are good, but it is always the jaw that gives away the fallacy of the scene. The lower jaw will fall away slightly when death is near, the most powerful muscles in the body finally releasing their hold. The actor-doctor will grab the jaw tightly and force it open to fit the blade of the scope and the long plastic tube into the airway. But in real life, the jaw falls away on its own and the paramedic or doctor or respiratory therapist only needs to position it out of his or her way gently, then let the scope do the rest. The slackness of the jaw is not something you can fake.

I pause for only a moment before falling on my knees to the pavement next to the boy's left side. David takes up a similar position at the boy's right hand and together, we work the patient. A bystander has secured his neck by placing her hands protectively around each side of his head and holding perfectly still. I see that she is holding the position correctly and thank God for small favors. "You've got his neck?" I ask her. If he survives, maybe he won't be paralyzed thanks in part to this good Samaritan.

"Yes, just like you taught me, Marianne," she responds, and I stop to look into her face for the first time. An image of this woman, leaning in close to take a blood pressure on a classmate in a high school classroom, flashes before me. Kathleen. Her name is Kathleen. She was my student the year before.

"Good job, Kathleen," I praise her, "thank you for helping." A man stands behind her, nearly in the ditch and watches, his eyes brimming with tears.

As I kneel beside the boy, I can hear the screech of sirens from the approaching Highway Patrol and volunteer fire personnel; we will have help very soon. The handheld radio in my pocket squawks incessantly; the helicopter will be approaching within a few minutes and they want to know where to land. I wish that I could turn the radio off, but instead, hand it to a firefighter who has appeared next to me. "Find a place where they can land!" I order.

I am used to working in relative quiet. I know, that sounds strange, but it's true. As paramedics, we are in charge of a scene, whether it's a car accident or a heart attack, we are in charge. When we respond to a call, we can say, "Turn the TV off, only one person talking at a time, don't yell at me, I'll leave." And most people will obey. We very rarely have the Hollywood drama queen portrayed as grief stricken young widows and devastated mothers whose sons have died in war. Most of the calls I responded to were quiet, sometimes unnaturally so.

So the murmuring and crying of the bystanders and the "whoosh, whoosh, whoosh" of cars and big rigs passing on the freeway half a mile away distract me. "Just let me work," I want to scream, but instead, I talk to the patient. I have this belief that if a patient hears his or her name during crisis, they will respond better and more quickly. They are transformed from "the patient" to Mary or Anthony and in this case, Jacob. They know we are working to save *them,* not just some unknown person we will forget when we drop them at the hospital.

"Jacob," I whisper above the noise all around us, "you've been injured and have a broken leg." I pull an IV setup from the trauma bag and pop the tubing together, attaching a large needle to the end of it. I wrap a tourniquet on the boy's upper arm and look for a vein in the crick of the elbow. "Ok Jacob, you're gonna feel a big poke in your arm." There, just where it should be, a fat, spongy vein appears and before I can hesitate, I swab the area with alcohol and stab my needle deep; a bright flash of blood appears in the catheter and I thread the inch long piece of plastic up the vein. David performs the same procedure on the other arm as well.

Someone, a firefighter probably, has secured a large plastic mask over the boy's face. When we arrived, the boy was breathing on his own and his airway had been surprisingly clear but, as we move to place a cervical collar on his neck, his body suddenly convulses and a plume of vomit erupts involuntarily from his mouth. I grab the portable suction machine that a firefighter has brought from the back of the ambulance and David sets up the intubation equipment from the large duffle bag that carries all of the supplies to assist respiration.

"Jacob, you've gotten a little sick but it's okay, we're gonna get that stuff out of your throat and help you breathe. Just relax," I tell him, although I know it doesn't matter if he relaxes or not. There's just something in the lack of response, the eyes now half open and unseeing, maybe after nearly four years on the job, I can see the spirit is no longer there.

We turn him on his left side, Kathleen still holding his

neck and head carefully. I suction his mouth and throat, waiting for the vomiting to stop. We roll him onto his back and I tell Kathleen she can let go for a minute; David is going to intubate and needs to be where she is.

"But, Marianne, you told me not to let go," Kathleen says. She doesn't move from her position but just stares at me.

"If we don't get his airway secure, Kathleen, he'll die. Do you remember, the first thing we always have to get is the airway?" The man behind her moves to touch her shoulder and she flinches when he makes contact.

"Kathy, let them handle it. It's their job," he says gently. She looks down at the boy and up to me again.

"Will you take care of him?" she asks me.

"I'll take care of him, I promise. You've done good, you don't have to stay." I tell her, hoping that the frustration and impatience I feel does not come through my voice. Finally, she releases her grip and stands, backing away until the man's arms find her and he encloses her into a tight hug.

The sound of the helicopter cuts the air. In a few minutes, Jacob will be on his way to the hospital. We work for several minutes to strap him to the backboard while David inserts a large tube into Jacob's throat and secures it with tape and attaches a large plastic ambu-bag to the end of the tube. We reassess Jacob and it is then that I see, sometime while we were being careful not to chip his teeth during the intubation and making sure that we wouldn't jostle him too much during transport, the light had gone from his eyes. We have failed. I take the ambu-bag attached to the tube in Jacob's throat and squeeze it firmly, one squeeze for every breath I take. I can feel eyes on me as I work and when I look up, find Kathleen and the man still standing close by, watching as Jacob is loaded onto a gurney.

"Kathleen, you don't have to stay. We'll take it from here," I tell her.

"He just went to get the mail," she whispers. "And he waited until the car passed." I look at her again and wonder what she is talking about. What mail? And then, I look to the ground and notice the mail again. He had gone to get the mail. "It was the second car; he was looking at the mail and the second car ..." she trails off and stares at Jacob again. "Marianne, will you go with him?" she asks.

"No," I say, "I can't fly on the helicopter."

"But, I know you'll take care of him, please go with him," tears fill her eyes and the man holds her tighter.

And suddenly, it hits me. My eyes follow hers and rest on Jacob; somewhere in his dark eyes and reddish-brown hair, I see Kathleen.

Kathleen is Jacob's mother.

In the field behind me, I hear the helicopter land a hundred feet away and its blades slow. Over the radio, David tells the flight nurse that the patient is ready, don't even bother slowing down, we'll bring him to you. A pack of firefighters begins to push the gurney; David takes the ambu-bag out of my hands and resumes compressing it every few seconds.

She finds me later, sitting on a cement bench outside the ambulance entrance to the hospital. They placed her son on a mechanical ventilator as soon he reached the hospital and despite the undivided attention of the best trauma surgeons in the far north state, his brain is too damaged and his body has given up. She has decided to donate his organs.

"He's healthy," she says, "and I figure maybe if his heart or lungs" she stops in mid sentence, her voice breaking as tears start to fall again.

"I know," I say, "I know," and even though I would like

to put an arm around her shoulders, I hold back.

"I did okay, though, didn't I?" she asks me. "I did everything you told me to, but …"

My heart skips a beat. I hold my breath and think. I wonder; did any of us do okay? How do we go on if we didn't do our best? How does a mother survive if she didn't do her best?

"You did perfect," I say. And she smiles.

DISNEYLAND

THE CALL CAME in the late afternoon of early June. A traffic collision, a rollover out on the freeway, beckoned. Martin and I responded almost immediately with lights and sirens. Mentally, I tick off the duties I must perform before we arrive at the scene: Dispatch the helicopter, make sure the fire department brings the rescue truck in case we have to extricate.

The accident, *but really, are they ever "accidents"?* filled both northbound lanes of the freeway just south of the overpass on the north side of town. On the emergency radio, the Highway Patrol officer on the scene advised us that we would not be able to reach the wreckage of the late-model pickup from the south; we would have to drive south, then cut through the oleanders in the median to get to the other side.

From the top of the overpass, I search the roadway below and find a line of cars that stretches into the horizon, stopped with impatient drivers, most unable to see the crumpled wreck of the teal blue Ford Ranger that has come to rest across the broken centerline of the road. Even from this distance, I can see that instead of heading north, the truck faces southwest, its windshield shattered. The crushed roof tells me the truck flipped at least once before finding its tires again.

The ambulance screams through the oblivious, southbound traffic of Interstate 5. In less than a mile, Martin pushes our heavy vehicle to nearly sixty-five miles an hour before finding a break in the tall, flowering bushes in the median and cutting to the northbound freeway lanes. He turns sharply at the line of cars steaming in the afternoon valley heat and drives the half mile in the dirt of the dry ditch beside the blacktop back up to the wreckage. Martin sweeps the ambulance around the first vehicle in the line of cars and stops in the middle of the road a few yards from the Ranger.

Martin glances at me as the ambulance stops; I stare at the chaos outside of my ambulance, at the dozens of people being good Samaritans, trying to do *something,* and I mentally count: one, two, three, four, five, six, seven, eight, nine, ten. *Just breathe,* I remind myself. I step from the ambulance and reach into the hidden side door of the patient compartment and grab the trauma bag. Martin steps up beside me and withdraws the airway bag and cardiac monitor. Together, we walk toward the wreckage and survey the scene methodically. Our patients, two girls, one in the vehicle, one lying in the middle of the road, wait for us as we brace ourselves for the coming chaos.

Her blond, shoulder-length hair falls over the headrest of the driver's seat in cascades of wheat; her mouth slack and her eyes, which I am sure were blue, are closed. Her head falls gently toward her right shoulder. Her long, thin arms rest at her side helplessly. She can't be more than eighteen or nineteen, if that, but that is all she will ever be. The man standing outside her door reaches into the cab of the truck and in a vain attempt to revive her, pushes *hard* on her chest repeatedly. With each compression, the seat behind her moves in, out, in, out. Remnants of a road trip—fast food restaurant bags, cassette tapes, empty soda bottles—litter the bench seat beside her. Piles of clothes, a curling iron, and a pair of oversized mouse ears attached to a dome shaped black cap form a mountain in the half seat behind her. Her best friend lies on the pavement a few feet from the truck. Neither had been wearing their seatbelt.

They had graduated from high school the week before somewhere in Oregon. The next day, they packed the truck and drove south to Disneyland for one last adventure as children before they were expected to take the responsibilities of adults. They were headed home, to work, to college, to boyfriends, when the driver, the girl with the wheat-blond hair, reached beneath her seat in search of a lost cassette tape. The gravel on the side of the freeway grabbed her tire but instead of riding it out, she pulled on the wheel *hard*. The small pickup overcorrected. Her best friend flew out the window and landed on the blacktop. She would live. But the girl with the wheat-blond hair and eyes the color of a Kansas summer sky, stayed in the truck and rolled with it. Her brain was unable to compensate for the pounding it took.

"I'll take her," Martin says and walks toward the dead girl in the truck.

My patient, a pretty teenaged cheerleader-type with deep brown hair, has come to rest on the hot pavement twenty feet away from the pickup truck. She is surrounded by several firefighters, each on his knees, cradling the girl in their own manner. One has his hands tightly cupped around her head, his large fingers forming a protective spider web around her face; one gently holds her right arm, tenderly wrapping a blood pressure cuff on the bare flesh of her upper arm; a third firefighter waits patiently at her left side, holding her hand while one of his colleagues places an oxygen mask over her mouth. I watch the men work for a moment and finally, although I feel like I will be intruding, step toward the girl and her fire-guardians.

When they see me approach, only the man with the blood pressure cuff falls away from her side and I slip in where he once kneeled. The firefighter tells me that even though she is unconscious, her blood pressure is good, her pulse steady. I remove the oxygen mask briefly and peer deep into the girl's mouth, glance at her pupils, check her pulse again, notice her breathing and conclude, that unless my three years in the field has been a lost education, she will live.

While the firefighters retrieve a backboard from the ambulance, I perform a quick physical exam, wrap a cervical collar around the girl's slim neck, start an IV, take another set of vitals: blood pressure, respirations, heart rate, oxygen saturation. I check her pupils periodically; if her brain decides to bleed, I want to know exactly when it happens. But her pupils stay small and even and I suspect her brain injury will only be the equivalent to a severe concussion.

The backboard arrives and I watch as several firefighters role her carefully to her side, slip the backboard under her body. When the back of her bare legs is exposed, I cringe at the redness developing on the pale skin and realize that the blacktop of the freeway has been cooking her while we worked on her. The firefighters role her halfway on her side, use a Velcro set of straps to secure her to the board, and place her on the gurney. The firefighters wheel my patient to the side of the ambulance for protection from the glaring sun and since she is stable and there are no procedures she needs that I can perform, we wait for the helicopter to retrieve her. I walk toward Martin and the dead girl in the truck to offer my assistance.

But Martin is not with the girl in the truck and contrary to every other time I have seen him with a patient, he has left her side. As I walk toward the truck, he watches me from his position near the ambulance. Two men I have never seen before stand at the edge of the girl's door, their strong arms alternately performing rudimentary CPR on her lifeless body. I glance at Martin and notice he has the microphone to the emergency radio in his hand; *he must be getting orders for a procedure or meds*, I think and walk toward him. He watches me approach and when I get within five feet, he whispers, "I'm calling it," and points to the radio with a latex-gloved hand. I nod my understanding, *he's getting permission from the hospital to pronounce his patient dead*, and glance back toward the men beside the dead girl.

The doctor on the other end of the radio listens as Martin gives the grim details of his patient's condition: She is pulseless and apneic, shows no signs of electrical activity on the cardiac monitor and both pupils are fixed and dilated. Bystanders have been performing CPR with the patient still sitting in her seat since the accident occurred; she's been down twenty minutes. The doctor knows the statistics better than Martin or I—less than one percent chance of recovery when cardiac arrest results from traumatic injury and that's only if CPR is performed properly, on a hard surface. The soft seat of the new truck provides no support, so essentially CPR on the girl sitting in her soft seat was in vain. Although the emergency department doctor patiently waits until the end of Martin's report, as soon as it is done, he sighs heavily into the radio and says, "Copy, Westside. Thank's for your report. Discontinue resuscitation and further treatment. I have time of death at 1744."

"Copy, 1744," Martin replaces the mike in its cradle and walks toward the men standing beside the dead girl's truck.

The firefighters who have been standing guard over my patient watch me closely as I approach her gurney, check her vitals again; she is stable, still unconscious, but breathing regularly. Her IV runs smoothly.

Martin reaches the truck and I watch as he speaks with the crowd that has gathered around the small Ford Ranger. His words are lost in the heavy traffic that speeds down the freeway on the opposite side of the oleanders but I imagine what he must be saying when he plants his long legs in a strong upside-down V, clasps his latexed-gloved hands in front of his chest, laces his fingers together, shakes his head side to side. *"I'm sorry,"* he seems to be saying, *"she never had a chance."* The men at her window continue their CPR, ignoring my partner. The crowd around Martin and the men shuffle and reposition; I watch the silent orchestration and wait. I've seen images like this before, but this time, there is something different. Normally, bystanders who happen on a fatal accident are repulsed; they may try to help the injured, but they shy away from the dead as quickly as possible. This crowd of five or six people moves closer to the girl in the front seat of the teal blue truck and when one of the men moves away from the window, I understand why. This girl does not look dead; she looks, instead, to be only sleeping. The change that happens to the body in the first thirty minutes or so of death has not happened to this girl and her injuries are internal, not gaping holes that announce certain death. And these people, who have been performing CPR and breathing into her lungs for the past twenty minutes, who may have even seen her driving on the road before the moment she reached under her seat for a lost cassette tape, do not believe that she is dead.

Martin moves to stand between his patient and the crowd, but suddenly, their voices, loud and demanding, stop Martin before he can find his way. "You have to do *something!*" One of the men yells at Martin. *"Do your fucking job!"* He moves threateningly toward Martin but my partner stands his ground, looking down at the man as he nears.

"She's not dead!" a woman behind Martin yells. And when he turns to address her, I imagine that he tells her, "Yes, she is," but his words are still so calm, that I cannot hear them.

The helicopter approaches and since we've decided to land it on the road a hundred feet from the truck, its engines drown out the crowd as they wave their arms and gesture wildly, yelling obscenities toward Martin. The firefighters wheel my patient toward the helicopter and as I walk past Martin and the crowd, their voices find me. "What do you mean you're not going to take her? The fucking helicopter's right there! We'll carry her to it! I'll carry her!" One of the men tells Martin. But Martin just shakes his head and stares at the ground.

The helicopter lifts off with my patient and carries with it, the resolve of the crowd. A firefighter finds a yellow plastic sheet and although the dead girl still sits upright in the front seat of the truck, the firefighter covers her body. The crowd disperses and eventually, a few drive their cars around the wreckage in the middle of the freeway and continue their journeys north. We wait until the sheriff-coroner arrives to secure the girl's body, then we load our gurney, put our bags and gear back into the ambulance.

Eventually, we will make it to the hospital, retrieve our backboard, and check on my patient. Eventually.

JENNIFER

LATE DECEMBER 1996

THE CALL CAME a little after four in the morning but for me, it started seven years prior.

Most calls have a clear beginning and end; for example, the call came at four in the morning and ended when we delivered the patient to the hospital or the helicopter or maybe, the patient refused treatment and we left them where we found them. And most calls are easy to detach from, even if we know the patient before the call, like my mom's friend Judy who would show up at ambulance quarters once or twice a week so I could check her blood pressure and put her on the cardiac monitor, "just to be sure," she would chime as I pressed the cardiac leads in place: *White over right, smoke over fire.* When placed correctly, white lead over the right shoulder, black lead over the left shoulder and red lead a few inches underneath, the leads can read the electrical activity in the heart. If needed, we can attach large sticky pads to thicker leads that send a shock directly across the cardiac muscle, stimulating the heart to resume its proper electrical activity, which tells the heart to pump blood throughout the body. But this call was not like most calls. And Jennifer was not just any patient. Jennifer, at one time, had been my best friend.

She had long red hair, thick like a horse's mane, that hadn't been cut since she was a young girl. On her petite frame, it nearly enveloped her when she leaned forward and when she sat down, an inch or two always caught under her bottom. She had tiny features and small hands and even after a baby, her tummy was flat and her waist narrow.

She had an easy laugh, even when her lips were coated with thick, deep red lipstick. And they always were. They matched the thick black lines that framed her narrow eyes and the long-dangly earrings that perpetually hung from her dainty lobes. She wasn't pretty in a conventional sense although pictures from her teen years revealed a soft skinned, smiling teen who could have surely been home-coming queen if she had run with the "in" crowd. But she hadn't and so she wasn't and fifteen years later, the drugs she had begun to smoke in her beautiful youth had caught up with her face and left it pockmarked and pasty white.

She was never without a boyfriend though, usually a young kid barely out of high school who had very little money and no job. They seemed to always ride bicycles instead of drive cars.

She always had a crowd around her and she always had a good job. She was a medical receptionist by trade; even after a night of drinking and smoking, she showed up to work on time and at least halfway alert, although more times than not, her eyes were half closed and she wore a crooked grin, slurring her words ever so slightly. And when one of her boyfriends used her as a punching bag, always aiming for one of her blue eyes, she would don an oversized pair of Jackie-O sunglasses and make breakfast for her kid and go to the grocery store and flirt with the bagboys as they helped her to her car. Smiling. She always kept the smile

The farmer found her on his way to his ranch, just before 5:00 on a cold December morning a few days before Christmas. He thought at first that she must have been a deer, struck dead by a passing car, her body thrown into the ditch like so many others before her. But as he slowed his pickup truck for the stop sign, she moved slightly, perhaps a leg or an arm, enough though, to catch his eye. He hesitated and finally slowed to a stop just a few yards from her body. He contemplated for a moment; should he get out and use his gun on the animal to stop its suffering? But it was cold outside of the warm cab of his truck and cows needed to be milked and he almost didn't have the heart to put the muzzle of a gun to a living creature. But if it was suffering.... He thought of his dog, the trusty Queensland Heeler that followed him all day as he worked. Would he want her to lie for hours suffering in the cold dark night?

He shifted the gear into park, grabbed a heavy coat from the bench beside him, and lifted the shotgun from the rack behind his head.

He pulled a shell from the inside pocket of his coat and shivered against the cold as he climbed out of the truck. He wondered how the animal had lived this long; the hypothermia should have set in by now and this burden wouldn't have fallen to his shoulders had the December air done its job, but it didn't matter. Because it hadn't and the animal was still alive and his heart ached at its suffering.

The shotgun was heavy as he rounded the corner of the truck bed but he balanced it in his hands lightly, ready to end the creature's misery as soon as he sited it. If he waited, he may not do it. The explosion of the shotgun would be deafening at this hour; the few neighbors in the rural area would wake and probably phone the sheriff, but it didn't matter, not much anyway. He would be held up answering their questions if someone happened to write down his license plate, but he doubted, as he glanced at the two houses closest to him, if anyone was awake this early.

He hesitated as he noticed a house, just across a small field, with lights blazing against the cold morning. Resolutely, he shook off his hesitation and turned back toward the dying doe. When he rounded the back of the truck, he raised the shotgun and in the instant before he would have pulled the trigger, he recognized the faint outline of a human foot. Heart racing, he dropped the barrel of the gun to his side and rushed forward. As he knelt down to her side to brush a tendril of hair from her cheek, a soft moan escaped her throat. He dropped the strand of chestnut red hair from his hand and rushed to the cab of his truck where he used his two-way radio to call for help.

We found her where the farmer had, face down in a shallow ditch, legs splayed and red hair nearly covering the entire top half of her body. She had walked a quarter mile or so from a nearby farmhouse, the one with its lights glowing brightly in the early morning darkness. The farmer had noticed it just before he had noticed her and the deputy sheriff who had gotten to the scene before us followed the fresh trail of blood from her body back to road in front of the white house with green trim. A large horse corral, square with thick white metal pipes framing a pasture, separated the house from Jennifer's body. The deputy had not moved her, but had instead, when he saw the gaping hole in her chest, inserted his index finger where the air escaped and probably saved her life. He was teased for the gesture later, and for the excitement he had let slip over the radio when he had reported her condition to us, "Unconscious female with a close range gunshot wound to the torso! It's a *sucking chest* wound!" The other deputies on duty and the dispatcher never let him forget that he let his guard down, something a cop was never supposed to do. When he had reported the sucking chest wound over the radio, my partner and I had rolled our eyes skyward and said simultaneously, "Rookie."

Martin, my partner, met the deputy before I had a chance to grab the airway and trauma bag. When I joined him on the side of the road a moment after we arrived, he and the deputy had stooped to examine the motionless body of the woman in the ditch.

"… gunshot wound, don't know how long she's been out here. Blood trail leads back to that house," the deputy jerked his head to the house with the glowing windows.

"Did you find the shooter?" Martin inquired.

"No, she was probably dumped. There's no one answering at the house and we don't know who she is. She's got track marks. She's probably just a junkie who pissed off the wrong boyfriend," the deputy said.

Martin grunted and reached for the woman's wrist to feel for a pulse. "Its faint, but its there," he said after a moment. "How far out's the helicopter?"

"Five minutes or so," I replied.

"We need a landing zone," Martin said, and stared at the deputy still by his side. His eyes seemed to will the deputy to move out of the way. The big man suddenly jerked back from the woman's body and he pushed himself up from the ground.

"Oh, yeah, yeah, sure. A landing zone," the deputy said.

I stepped closer to the ditch and waited for the deputy to move out of my way. I dropped the airway and trauma bags beside Martin and for the first time, found myself staring at the woman in the ditch.

It was the hair that I recognized first; even in the early morning darkness, the chestnut mane was unmistakable.

"Her name's Jennifer," I said. Martin swept her hair away from her body and revealed an ugly wound the size of a dinner plate across her abdomen and torso.

"What?" Martin asked me.

"Her name's Jennifer," I repeated.

"You know her?" the deputy who had reappeared at my side asked.

"Yes. She's … was … I knew her, a long time ago."

Martin stopped the evaluation of her body and stared at me for several seconds. "You gonna be okay?" he asked.

"Mm-hmm," I muttered. For a moment or more, I stood and watched Martin work. Finally, my brain cleared. "She's got a kid. A boy named Parker. She lives in town. And a sister named Katie. She lives in town too. Over on Eighth Street."

The cold gravel on the side of the road dug into my knees as I knelt beside her. Martin worked to stabilize her; a firefighter retrieved the backboard from the ambulance. We stemmed the flow of blood with several large bandages; I wiped blood from her chest and stomach. I pushed her long hair from her face and cleared the heavy makeup that had run to the ridge above her cheeks. Just before the helicopter landed, we rolled her to the backboard, secured her body so she wouldn't fall, and wrapped a heavy blanket around her naked form.

I saw her a few summers ago; the first time in nearly a decade. She had been clean for a few years and had managed to hold a job long enough to be the supervisor of a local thrift shop. It was eight to five, Monday through Friday. Honest, respectable work. Her hair was a little shorter than I remember, but at nearly forty-five, she still had the same petite frame, open smile, and pretty blue eyes. The years had been kinder to her since that morning just before Christmas in 1996; the lines around her eyes are not as deep as I remember and the distrust of the world had left her gaze.

She engulfs me in a giant hug and a flash of her, lying in the ditch, hits me when her arms circle me. "How've you been?" she asks.

"I'm good," I reply. "Just working, married."

"You married the cop, right?" She asks and I wonder how she knows about my husband.

"Yes, Matt," I confirm. "You're doing well?" I ask but suddenly, I realize I don't want to know the answer to my question. I move away and just out of her reach.

"I'm great, clean. First time in a long time." The smile and clear eyes told me that before she had spoken, but she is proud of it, of what she has come from, to where she is now. "I've been here for three years and now I run the place. Isn't that a kick?" she asks.

"That's fantastic," I tell her, and it really is.

She tells me about the boyfriend she has been dating for a year or two, a nice guy, she says. Not like all the others. He has a good job and treats her well. Her son, Parker, whose diapers I used to change, is twenty years old now. No, he isn't in college, but he's doing okay. Ready to say goodbye, I move away from my old friend and say, "I'll call you soon," even though I know I won't. Her posture changes suddenly and she steps toward me and whispers, "You know I got shot, didn't you?"

"Jennifer—" I stammer.

"You didn't know?" she asks me. I search her bright blue eyes. "Or have I seen you since then? I lost, like, a year."

"At Grace's wedding, you showed me the scar," I remind her. "And Jennifer, I was there. When you were shot, I was the paramedic."

She steps back from me and tears spring to her eyes. "You were there," she asks. "You were the one?"

"My partner and I, yes. I was on the ambulance," I tell her.

"You saved my life," she says, and hugs me again. Her tears fall on my shirt and when she finally pulls away from me, a dull haze has replaced the light that had been in her eyes a few minutes ago. Her lipstick is smudged a little and her thick mascara slides down her pale cheeks. Her expression tells me that she knows what I have seen, how I have seen her and the embarrassment and shame come like a wave over her face. I try to see the Jennifer in front of me, but suddenly, I am back on the side of the road on a cold December morning in 1996, and Jennifer is naked, lying in the ditch.

BREATHE

THE CALL CAME a little after 8:00 on a warm summer night; a female with shortness of breath. The sun had already set but the heat of the valley, which stays into the early morning hours, still clung to the trees and streets. The air becomes heavy in late June–early July every year in the valley. It's predictable that way. On February 1, it always rains and come July, the heat never goes away.

A little after 8:00, most of the television sets in the newer working class neighborhood just north of town were set to baseball. The season was nearing its fourth month lull but most of the men and a few women in town, nearly every evening, watched the A's and Giants anyway. The Giants were in the middle of a ten-game losing streak and the A's weren't doing much better; each would end the 1996 season with less than 50 percent of their games won, the glory of the 1989 season and the World Series distant memories.

But on this night, there was still hope for the season.

The woman standing on the sidewalk in front of the small yard stares at me through my window. I've seen this look before and know, before I open the ambulance door and step to the curb, whatever she has to tell me will be bad. The ambulance rolls to a stop. Ed, my temporary partner, sits behind the steering wheel and doesn't see the woman. And he doesn't understand when I thrust the door open, reach into the back of the ambulance, grab my bag, and run. The woman, a pretty Latina in her early thirties with shoulder length wavy hair and dark eyes, pulls me with her toward a small stucco house.

"The baby was breathing a minute ago," the woman tells me as we enter her neat, well-kept bungalow.

"Baby, what baby?" I ask stupidly. She drags me down a short, dark hallway.

"The baby!" she repeats and as we come to the end of the hallway, she pushes a door open and shows me: the baby.

The bathroom is small, with just enough room for a pedestal sink, a narrow tub, and toilet. The walls are pale cream, probably the same color the house was originally painted ten years before. A small rug hides the square of linoleum that covers the floor.

A woman, somewhere approaching thirty years old but not quite there, sits on the toilet, her pants pushed down to the floor and a large tent-like red cotton top pulled up to expose a swollen belly. She could be the twin of the woman who met me in the yard, except her face is pale, eyes sunken into fleshy cheeks. Her hair is pulled into a ponytail. Cupped in her hands, the smallest human I have ever seen rests.

"She was breathing just a minute ago," the woman on the toilet tells me.

I fall to my knees on the soft rug in front of the toilet. My airway bag is forgotten in the hallway along with the woman who met me outside. Without words, the mother hands the baby to me.

The baby girl fits easily into my hands, with her soft fuzzy head resting on my left palm and her feet dangling just past the tips of my fingers. A faint echo of blood taints her skin slightly pink. Regardless, she is pale, with soft brown hair, her lips slightly blue. Her eyes are tightly closed.

My lips find the baby's mouth and nose. I cover the blue skin, make a seal with my own mouth, and breathe, breathe. Two of my fingers search for the spot on the baby where the heart should be, between the nipples and down, just an inch or so. I examine the baby as I compress the tiny chest quickly, one, two, three, four, five. Breathe, breathe. Compress one, two, three, four, five. Breathe, breathe. She has ten fingers and ten toes and weighs only one or two pounds; too tiny to be born over a toilet. But even if she had not been small, she is still not perfect.

Her mother sits on the toilet, watching me. Blood from the birth has pooled around the base of the toilet and she must have caught her daughter with her own hands before the baby girl fell into the bowl. Large, red handprints paint the cream walls behind and in front of the toilet. The umbilical cord is still attached so I try to keep the baby at the same level as the mother's still-swollen belly to prevent the baby's blood from flowing back into the mother's womb.

"Is she going to be alright," the mother asks.

"I'm doing everything I can for her," breathe, breathe. Compress one, two, three, four, five.

"But she'll be alright?"

"What's your name?" breathe, breathe. Compress one, two, three, four, five.

"Anna," she replies.

"When is your due date, Anna?" breathe, breathe. Compress one, two, three, four, five.

"I don't know." She stares at her daughter, watches me as I breathe softly into her lungs.

"Who's your doctor?" breathe, breathe. Compress one, two, three, four, five.

"I don't have one," worry fills her voice.

"She can't be pregnant," Anna's sister says from the hall-way. I stop CPR for a brief moment and stare at the woman, the baby cradled in my hands. "I mean, she's never even had sex, she's never had a boyfriend."

Breathe, breathe. Compress one, two, three, four, five. In the hallway, Ed pushes his way through several family members who have gathered at the door.

"What the fuck?"

"I need the OB kit and see if we have a tube small enough for her. She's got a bunch of crap in her throat but she was breathing just before we got here," breathe, breathe. Compress one, two, three, four, five.

"The OB kit?" his gaze follows the umbilical cord from the mother to the baby and he sees what I have been hiding from the mother. "Oh Jesus." He drops the trauma bag and cardiac monitor; his footfalls thump heavily on the carpeted hallway as he runs toward the ambulance. Breathe, breathe. Compress one, two, three, four, five.

My mind races to organize what procedures the little girl cupped in my hands needs but I get stuck on the prime mantra I learned in paramedic school: Airway, breathing, circulation, the ABC's of emergency medicine. I must take care of the ABC's.

Compress one, two, three, four, five. In medicine, there are priorities that cannot be overlooked. Priority one is airway. If the airway is blocked, unblock it. If the airway has the likelihood to become compromised, put a tube in it to protect it. Take care of the airway first, then move on to breathing. If the patient's breathing has stopped, breathe for them. If the patient's lungs are damaged, give them medicine to fix them. And finally, after the airway and breathing are taken care of, check circulation. If the heart has stopped beating, compress it and give medications to restart it. If the patient is bleeding profusely, stem the flow of blood. Airway, breathing, circulation: The building blocks of emergency medicine. It is my job to fix what is broken.

My mind is suddenly clear and focused. I have one singular goal; secure the airway. I need help, though, because the baby's airway is full of mucous and my hands are occupied with the continuous motion of chest compressions. The airway is not secure. I must get free of the mother, who is still attached to the baby via umbilical cord. I need to get to my ambulance, where I have tools and medicine that will help me secure the airway. It feels like Ed has been gone a lifetime and I cannot leave my patient to find him and the OB kit I need. Breathe, breathe. Compress one, two, three, four, five. I am trapped in the small bathroom with the blood soaked bath mats and the blood stained walls.

Anna's sister watches me from the hall. I realize I have forgotten to tell Ed to call the helicopter. I turn my gaze to the hallway. "What's your name?" I ask Anna's sister. Breathe, breathe. Compress one, two, three, four, five.

"Me? Laura," she replies.

"Ok Laura, can you do me a favor?" Breathe, breathe. Compress one, two, three, four, five. She nods her head. "Can you get me a pair of scissors and a couple of shoelaces?" Breathe. Breathe.

"Shoelaces?"

"Yes, just any shoelaces, please, hurry. And I need a phone." Breathe, breathe. My radio is not working in the house and I need to talk to Dispatch.

"Don't you have that stuff," she asks me accusingly.

"I do, but it's in my ambulance and I don't have time to wait," breathe, breathe. Compress one, two, three, four, five. "Bring me the phone first." Breathe, breathe.

Laura returns a moment later with a cordless telephone.

She pushes it toward me. "Can you dial a number for me?" Breathe, breathe. Compress one, two, three, four, five. "Dial 1-800-555-7300. Ask for ambulance dispatch. Tell them it's an emergency." Breathe, breathe. In the hallway, Laura speaks into the phone.

"They want to talk to you," Laura pushes the phone toward me again.

"Laura, I need you to talk to them for me. Can you do that?" Breathe, breathe. Compress one, two, three, four, five.

"I guess," she hesitates and returns the phone to her ear. It will have to do.

"Tell them Westside is on a call in Orland. CPR in progress on an infant. Dispatch the helicopter." Breathe, breathe. Thirty seconds pass as Laura speaks into the phone. Breathe, breathe. Compress one, two, three, four, five.

"They think it's a prank," Laura says.

"Ask the dispatcher his name," I instruct. She speaks quietly into the phone again.

"Robby, he says he's a dispatcher." *Robby, thank god. He and I were close friends.*

"Put the phone up to my ear," I tell her. Breathe, breathe. Compress one, two, three, four, five. Laura steps into the bathroom and places the phone a few inches from my ear. "Robby, its Marianne. My radio isn't working," breathe, breathe. Compress one, two, three, four, five.

"What's goin' on out there?" Robby asks.

"I need the helicopter and fire department," breathe, breathe. Compress one, two, three, four, five.

"Are you doing CPR?" he asks me. He must have heard the rhythmic mantra.

"Yes, I've got a mom and newborn. Mom is good but baby is ..." breathe, breathe. Compress one, two, three, four, five. "Blue and unresponsive. She's been down about five minutes." Breathe, breathe. Compress one, two, three, four, five.

Robby suddenly shifts, a noticeable drop in his voice tells me he understands the situation. As I listen, tones on the other end of the phone signal the helicopter dispatch. "Enloe Flightcare, medical emergency at 842 Almond Street, Orland. Paramedics on scene, CPR in progress." Breathe, breathe. Compress one, two, three, four, five. "Marianne, they're in route. Fire has also been dispatched. Anything else I can do for you?" Breathe, breathe.

"Gotta go, Robby. Thanks." I push the phone away with the side of my head and turn toward Laura. "Shoelaces? And scissors?" Breathe, breathe. Compress one, two, three, four, five. Laura turns and runs out of sight.

"Is she gonna be OK?" Anna asks. Tears stream down her face, mixing with the blood on her thighs.

"I don't know, Anna. She's pretty small," breathe, breathe. Compress one, two, three, four, five. "How are you feeling?" She has lost a lot of blood, more than I've seen on any of the other deliveries I witnessed.

"I'm OK. I just had to go to the bathroom," Anna explains.

"You felt pressure?" Breathe, breathe. Compress one, two, three, four, five.

"Mmhmm," she nods.

"And when you pushed?" Breathe, breathe. Compress one, two, three, four, five.

"She just ... came out. I caught her."

"Did she fall into the water?" Breathe, breathe. Compress one, two, three, four, five.

"No, almost, but I caught her. Her name's Christina. I'm gonna name her Christina." Hope fills her eyes as she watches me. Christina. Her name is Christina. Of Christ. I know; my middle name is Christine. Breathe, breathe.

Compress one, two, three, four, five.

Laura returns with an old pair of tennis shoes that may have been white when they were new. "Do they have to be clean?" She asks me.

"No, just take them out of the shoes and give them to me," breathe, breathe. Compress one, two, three, four, five. "Anna, I need to take Christina to the ambulance so I can treat her better, OK?" Breathe, breathe. Sirens in the distance tell me the fire department is coming; help is on the way. Anna and Laura watch me closely as I cradle Christina in my left hand; if I wanted, I could nearly hide the baby girl between my hands. "I need your help, Laura. I need you to take one of those shoelaces and tie it as close to the baby's tummy as you can." Breathe, breathe. Compress one, two, three, four, five. Laura steps into the bathroom and I hold the baby out toward her, my fingers careful not to leave her chest. The rhythm of the compressions makes the baby's belly jiggle slightly against the palm of my hand. When I raise my hand from Christina's tummy so Laura can tie the shoelace, she gasps.

"Oh my God!" Laura cries. Fresh tears fill her eyes.

"It's OK, the doctors can fix that." Breathe, breathe. Compress one, two, three, four, five. But I don't know if they can fix that, or even what *that* is. Where smooth, pink skin should cover her tummy, the baby only has a thin, dark red layer of pseudo-skin. Through the pseudo-skin, faint outlines of large intestine, stomach and blood vessels are visible. Breathe, breathe. Compress one, two, three, four, five. "Wrap the shoelace around the cord right by her tummy." Laura holds the shoelace tenderly, her hands shaking and tears trailing her cheeks. She wraps the lace around the thick, white cord, ties a loose knot, and pulls gently. "You gotta pull tight, make sure the knot is good and pull." Breathe, breathe. Compress one, two, three, four, five. Laura repositions the lace and ties the knot again. She pulls the lace tight, squeezing the cord closed.

"Good job," breathe, breathe. "Ok, now take the other lace and tie it just the same way a few inches away from the first knot." Compress one, two, three, four, five. This time, she grasps the cord and pulls the knot tight on the first try. "Good. The scissors?" Breathe, breathe. Laura finds the scissors and pushes them toward me. Compress one, two, three, four, five. "You're gonna have to do it, Laura."

"Won't it hurt the baby?" Laura asks, wide-eyed and pale.

"Nope, she won't feel a thing. Just hold the cord and cut between the two knots. It'll be tough, like a garden hose, so cut hard." Breathe, breathe. Compress one, two, three, four, five.

"Will it hurt, Anna?" Laura asks her sister.

"Just cut, Laura."

"Mija, please, cut it," Anna pleads with her sister. Laura takes the cord in her hand and with the scissor, cuts cleanly through.

Breathe, breathe. Compress one, two, three, four, five.

Free. I am finally free to carry the baby Christina to the ambulance. My partner, Ed, passes me in the hall as I walk-run toward the ambulance.

"Where are you going?" Ed asks me.

Breathe, breathe. Compress one, two, three, four, five.

"To the ambulance. I need to intubate her and get an IV." Compress one, two, three, four, five. "Grab the monitor and the bags." I feel Ed staring at me as I walk out of the house. A police car has arrived and just behind, the first fire truck appears. The warm summer night has become a practice in ordered chaos and strobe light spectacle in the few minutes I was inside the house. A young, thin firefighter wearing firefighting turnout pants, heavy boots, and a

white t-shirt meets me at the front door of the small bungalow. Breathe, breathe. Compress one, two, three, four, five.

"What 'cha got?" he asks. I've seen him on calls before.
He is a certified emergency medical technician and carries
a bag with oxygen, stethoscope, and blood pressure cuff.

"Newborn not breathing. Mom needs to be watched.
Can you stay with her?" Breathe, breathe. Compress one,
two, three, four, five.

"Sure, she inside?"

"Yeah, Ed's in there. She's in the bathroom," breathe,
breathe. "Hey, watch her pressure, she's lost a lot of blood."
Compress one, two, three, four, five.

"Will do," the firefighter confirms.

It feels like my fingers have been working forever, like
the wings of a hummingbird, on the tiny life cradled in
my hands. My ambulance—home at times like this, the
most comfortable place for me to be—waits just beyond
the parched lawn of the bungalow and I nearly sprint toward its bright lights. Breathe, breathe. I feel Ed, hear the
jingle of his ever-present ring of keys, close behind me.
Steve Monk, the police officer who just arrived, opens the
rear ambulance double doors. He is a paramedic also and
works for our ambulance part-time. I climb into the back
of the ambulance and carefully place the baby on the bench
seat beside the gurney. I sit on the gurney in front of her.
Breathe, breathe. Compress one, two, three, four, five.

Ed jerks the side door of the ambulance open and shoves
the medical bags into the cubby hidden behind the steel
walls of the patient compartment. He clamors up the steps,
his shaved head barely scraping the ceiling, and kicks tubing and plastic bags from beneath his feet.

"I can't find the fucking OB kit. Or a tube to intubate
her. What size do you think she would take?" Ed searches
through another cabinet randomly tossing oxygen masks,

bags of saline, and IV catheters to the floor. A box of latex gloves flies through the open divider to the cab of the ambulance.

Breathe, breathe. Compress one, two, three, four, five.

"The OB kit should be under the shelves, in the bottom of the cabinet. Its in a box," breathe, breathe.

Steve Monk stands outside the ambulance, just beyond the doors, and watches us work. Pale pink skin shines through his light brown hair, lights from the ambulance highlighting the baldness that is only a few years away. He seems small standing in the street, several feet below where I sit on the gurney. His uniform hangs slightly from his frame even though I know it is fairly new and he hasn't lost any weight recently. And he's as tall as I am, nearly 5'8", with a little paunch at his lower belly, not much, but enough to show through the ill fitting uniform shirt. Breathe, breathe. Compress one, two, three, four, five. I must look flustered or tired or beat, something, because he suddenly steps toward the ambulance.

"Can I help?" Steve asks, his thick mustache twitching, his brown-green eyes riveted on the baby. I nod my head between breaths, "yes, please, yes." He steps into the ambulance and sits next to me on the gurney. It's cramped inside the patient compartment of the ambulance, but since Ed has been occupied trying to find supplies, I need a second pair of hands. Breathe, breathe. Compress one, two, three, four, five.

"I'm gonna need a line on her, can you search for a vein?" I ask Steve.

Ed abruptly stops throwing sheets and blankets from the cabinet. Breathe, breathe. Compress one, two, three, four, five.

"Marianne, do you want me to take over CPR?" Ed asks hopefully. "You know where the OB kit is." He's right,

I do, but CPR on an infant is a one-person job; babies are too small to have more than one person compressing their chests like a hummingbird on a hot summer day and breathing into their tiny mouths. And I have already been exposed to this baby and her mother's blood and birthing fluids. I will be required to be tested for HIV, hepatitis, and sexually transmitted infections like herpes, gonorrhea, and chlamydia; there is no reason for Ed to be exposed also.

"No, find an oxygen mask small enough for her first, then we'll switch," breathe, breathe. Compress one, two, three, four, five. "Does the fire department know the helicopter is coming?"

"They're setting up a landing zone in a field across the street," Steve responds.

Over the radio, Neil, the flight nurse on the helicopter, talks to dispatch. We have been ignoring his calls for several minutes.

"Enloe Dispatch, Westside is not responding to radio. Do you have an update on the patient?" Neil asks. Breathe, breathe. Compress one, two, three, four, five.

"Negative Flightcare, last contact was 2037, CPR in progress." Robby the dispatcher responds.

"Copy, we'll contact fire on scene. What channel is Orland Fire?"

"Copy, Flightcare. Orland Fire is available on channel two," Robby replies.

"Copy. ETA three minutes," Neil signs off. Behind me, Ed digs in the airway bag, tossing equipment much too large for the baby cradled in my hands, to the floor.

"The pediatric masks and bag are on the top shelf, over the suction," I snap. Breathe, breathe. Compress one, two, three, four, five. Finally, he snags a tiny plastic mask and ambu-bag (a semi-rigid plastic bag that is used to ventilate), and fits them together. I bend once more to the miniature mouth and nose and *breathe, breathe.* Ed slips the plastic mask over the baby girl's face and begins to squeeze the ambu-bag every few seconds. Steve takes over compressions while we reposition. Ed takes my place in front of the baby while I stretch my legs across the gurney and plant my feet in the narrow space on the other side. I open a cabinet down by the floor and pluck a white, cardboard box from its depths. Large black letters printed across the top, "OB GYN," confirm what it is. I rip it open and extract a lemon-sized suction bulb. I move back to the baby and push my way toward her head.

"Lemme see her," I order. Ed removes the oxygen mask and I plunge the bulb's long suction tube deep into her mouth. "We gotta get this crap out of her mouth and lungs," I say as I suction. I take a cloth and clean the bulb while Ed squeezes the ambu-bag over her face again. He moves the mask and I plunge the bulb into the baby's throat again; I would use the mechanical suction, but there are no tubes small enough to fit in her throat and the suction power of the mechanical device would most likely collapse her fragile lungs.

"Sonovabitch," I mutter quietly. "I can't see anything." I remove the bulb again and let Ed replace the oxygen mask; he compresses the ambu-bag rhythmically while Steve compresses the baby's tiny chest. "She's too small," I say, defeated.

The sound of the approaching helicopter fills the warm night air. The "thwup, thwup" of the bird momentarily hypnotizes me.

"Do you want to start an IV?" Steve reminds me. "We can start meds if she's got a line." His pale face glistens with sweat and he looks tired, dark moons underlining his brown eyes. I wonder how long we have been working on the baby.

"Yes, an IV," I reply, shaken from my reverie. I examine the baby's forehead, a prime spot on newborns for IVs, but see nothing; it is smooth and surprisingly pink. And then I remember the blood in the bathroom. Her skin is still tinted from the blood of her birth. "Does she have anything on her legs or arms we could tap? Maybe the top of her foot?"

Steve, still compressing her chest and with the best view of her body, glances over the tiny body briefly.

"Maybe her foot," he confirms.

We apply a tourniquet to her bird-like leg and watch for the vein to appear. A small blue line appears just below her ankle, on the top of her foot. Before it disappears, I swab it with alcohol and stab it with the smallest butterfly needle we carry. I wait for the telltale flash of blood in the catheter signaling success, but it never comes and I know my one shot at an IV is gone. My mind races, running through the possibilities left. If we can get the phlegm and fluid out of her lungs, we can intubate and give her medication that way. Maybe we can find another vein. Or maybe, we can do an intraosseous line.

There are procedures you hope you will never be forced do in the field. Some procedures, like decompressing a collapsed lung, doing a cricothyrotomy, or cardioverting an athlete and saving him or her from a lethal cardiac rhythm, are exciting because usually, they work. My favorite is waking a diabetic from an insulin overdose. One minute, the grim reaper is knocking on the door, the next, the person is watching the 49ers on the big screen saying, "nope, I'm good, don't need to go to the hospital." Those days, those calls - you know you've saved a life. You've done your job.

But there is nothing good about being forced to do an intraosseous line.

Doing an intraosseous in the field means several things: One, the patient is a child. Two, the child is critically ill or injured. And three, all other options have failed and there-fore, you have failed. In paramedic school, we practiced on detached chicken legs to learn how to perform an intraos-seous; it was the only time in school we got to touch real flesh that didn't belong to one of our classmates.

There is a trick to performing an intraosseous line on a baby; it begins with finding the correct spot on the upper shin, just below the knee. It is the spot where the bone has not been fully formed yet. On a chicken leg, it is the spot just below the head of the leg, at the top of the narrow shaft of leg. A special needle-catheter with a thick shaft of steel at its core, attached to thick plastic handles so the technician can push through the bone, is used to perform an intraos-seous. The needle is an inch to an inch and a half long. The trick is, the correct spot must be punctured through the layer of bone at the top of the leg into the marrow canal below, without puncturing the back of the bone and com-ing out the other side. On a child two or three years old, the trick isn't so hard. But on a one- or two-pound infant, whose leg isn't any bigger than a fat permanent marker, the trick is nearly impossible.

I check once more for an alternate vein. Protocol tells me I must make two attempts to start an IV before initiat-ing the intraosseous procedure, but a quick examination confirms that there are no viable veins for a second attempt at the more conventional and standard IV.

"We need to do an intraosseous," I inform the medics. Ed continues to breath for the baby and Steve compresses her chest without rest. I gather the appropriate equipment: intraosseous needle, IV setup, alcohol swab, syringe filled with saline, bandages, tape.

"Have you ever done an intraosseous?" Steve asks me.

"No," I say. "Only in school."

"I have, once. I'm in position, do you want me to do it?"

His position at the foot of the baby provides the perfect placement for the procedure.

Without hesitation, I hand him the equipment. The three of us, Ed, Steve and I, reposition again. This time, I take the ambu-bag, which I am closest to, Ed begins compressions on the baby's chest, and Steve preps the baby's leg for the intraosseous. I watch as he cleans the leg with alcohol, feels for the correct spot, pierces the mottled skin below the baby's right knee. A soft "pop" echoes in the ambulance as the needle-catheter enters the marrow cavity. Steve removes the inner shaft of the needle, which drove the needle into the bone, leaving in place the needle-catheter with thick wings. He attaches the syringe to the catheter. To make sure he has placed the catheter in the correct space he gently pulls on the syringe's plunger. When no blood appears, he shoots a small amount of saline through the catheter. If the saline enters easily and does not infiltrate the skin around the site or on the other side of the leg, we have succeeded. If not, we have one more leg on which to try the procedure.

"I think its good," Steve says after a few seconds.

"Me too," I agree. "Push a little more saline and see what it does."

A blond figure appears at the back of the ambulance, beyond the open doors. *"How did he get here so fast?"* I wonder to myself and then realize the night air is suddenly quiet. Neil's long blond hair is disheveled, wind swept, and I wonder if he was standing on the skid of the helicopter when it landed, like I had seen others do. It was like they couldn't wait to get to the scene, care for the patient. Often, when the helicopter descended on a scene, Mike or Neil or Donna would begin to lean out the side of the aircraft, holding onto a long strap with one arm, so they didn't plummet to the ground. They are all thin, Neil and

Donna relatively short, so they don't throw off the balance of the bird. I had seen Mike stand on the helicopter's skid from fifty feet up and then jump a few feet before the bird had a chance to land. It took only one bad crash in 2001 in Butte Meadows, when the pilot was killed and Mike was injured, to stop the practice. But tonight, they had landed safely and Neil, the medic on the helicopter, stared at the baby on the bench seat and waited while Steve pushed fluid through the tiny catheter buried in her leg. Normally jovial and laid back, Neil's face tensed and pinched as he assessed the baby. He didn't say anything to us for nearly a minute. He broke his statuesque posture and moved to take over the attempt to give the infant oxygen.

We work her for another thirty minutes in the back of the ambulance. The phlegm and fluid in her lungs finally loosens and Neil is able to insert a tube into her throat. He gives her epinephrine and atropine, enough to revive a horse, he says, and for a few minutes, the electrical currents in her heart begin to flutter. In the end, it is not enough.

I see Neil a few days later, sitting just inside the ambulance bay doors at the desk where we can write our reports. He's quiet and pensive; it is the first time I've ever seen him alone. He leans back in his chair, laces his fingers behind his head, when I stop to say hello.

"How you doin'?" he asks me. And I know what he means.

"I'm okay. The mom tested negative for HIV and STDs, so, I should be okay." I shuffle my feet and play with the pen in my hand. "I'm good, though. You know?"

"Yeah," he says, and I wonder if I've convinced him.

"You doin' okay?" I ask him.

He nods his head quickly and although he stares straight toward me, I can see that his thoughts are elsewhere. "I just keep thinking, *If we could have gotten that crap out of her lungs, we could have given her meds and she'd've made it.'"*

"Yeah, I don't know," I say, "she had other things going on, and she was so small. ..." I try to comfort him but the confusion and hurt in his eyes tells me I am only salting the wound.

"I don't know," he says. His hands fall from his hair and he leans forward in his chair. "How'd you do it?" he asks me suddenly. His eyes sharpen and focus on me.

"What do you mean?"

"Man, I wanted so bad to just—to just—put my mouth over that baby's mouth and suck that crap out of her lungs."

"Me too," I say. The click of the pen, in, out, in, out, echoes in the small space of the makeshift office. My feet feel heavy and I want to move, but can't.

"But, you did do it," he says to me.

"I ..." and I stop.

"How did you do that? I've never done mouth to mouth before," he nearly cries. And I realize the look in his eye, the loneliness and desperation of his voice. He has been a medic much longer than I, was one of the first medics on the helicopter in the early '80s, and still, he hesitated in his duty when I had not.

"I didn't think about it," I say, trying to assuage his guilt. And it's true, I didn't.

"Exactly," he says, and I watch him as he walks down the long hallway, his soft blond hair falling gently across his defeated shoulders.

THE TOOTHACHE

IN PARAMEDIC SCHOOL and in the field, instructors and veteran medics downplay the inherent stress of the job. Instructors will say, "As long as you know your job, you'll do fine. Just always know your job," and continue innocuous demonstrations such as how to stab an orange with a two-inch needle or how to start an IV on a life-sized plastic arm. And veterans, those people who have been in the field at least ten years or so, will laugh when you ask, "So, what's the worst part of the job?" They don't laugh because they think its funny; they laugh because if they knew, they wouldn't be doing the job. But stress is the reason people leave so quickly, why the burnout rate for a paramedic is less than ten years. Why paramedics are more likely than the average person to have an affair, to commit suicide, and to use illicit drugs. It's getting better; in the mid-1990s, the burnout rate stood right around four years.

It comes from all sides in prehospital emergency medicine. The patient yells in pain; the family yells because you didn't get there quick enough; doctors glare and occasionally, when you've really screwed up, they tell you to leave. "Get the hell out of my hospital before you kill someone!" Screaming doctors don't cause the most stress; the most stress often comes from the unexpected and unlikely sources. When you are a paramedic, the most stress comes from the perfectly mundane. I often ask paramedics who have left the field, "why, why did you leave"? And they tell me stories of broken families, long hours, the managers who expected miracles all day, every day, and the one call—that final call—when they realized they were done.

The call came at 3:00 a.m. on a frigid winter morning in March 1997. A thirty-four-year-old man with an address just up the block from ambulance quarters, in run-down apartments we are all too familiar with, has a toothache. It's my call and I wonder today, would this have been my breaking point if the call rotation had fallen to my partner? Would I still be working on the ambulance? But the rotation had fallen to me and the toothache was mine.

It takes only a minute from quarters to reach the low-income apartments where the man with the toothache lives. My eyes are still swollen with sleep and my boots are just barely zipped when I spot a Latino man standing on the sidewalk outside the apartments. The man, wearing a thin, worn multi-colored 1970s polyester coat, faded blue jeans, and work boots, bows his head as the lights of our ambulance flash in his dark brown eyes. A girl, no more than eight or nine years old, stands next to him. They are waiting for us, even though it's nearly freezing and the girl is wearing only shorts, a thin shirt, and flip-flops. Her dark, wavy hair falls to her shoulders and makes a deep contrast to the pale pink t-shirt with the giant purple cartoon dinosaur on the front. The resemblance between the two is noticeable. She has his deep-set eyes and if the man ever let his hair grow out, it would be identical to his daughter's.

I roll the window down as the ambulance nears the curb. "Did you call the ambulance?" I ask the father. He looks alarmed and glances at the girl.

"Yes, my papa. His tooth hurts." The girl wraps her arms around her body and tries to capture some of the heat that escapes into the frigid air. The father nods quickly in confirmation.

"And you want to go to the hospital?" I can feel my partner, David, rustling behind the driver's seat. He's impatient and would rather be sleeping. And he forgot his Diet Coke. Before leaving quarters, on every call, David grabs a Diet Coke on his way out. On this call, he forgot.

The girl speaks quietly in Spanish to her father. He leans in to hear her, then straightens up and nods. Yes, he wants to go to the hospital.

An involuntary sigh escapes my lips as I open the passenger door and motion for them to follow me. Warm air and bright lights flood the girl as I open the double doors at the back of the ambulance. I wait for her to climb into the giant box, then over the gurney and onto a seat tucked away between the cabinets filled with blankets and medication and plastic tubing. Her father follows, taking his place on the gurney. He sits upright, with his feet still on the ambulance floor and his hands in the pockets of his coat. I pull the doors of the ambulance closed behind me and find the warm bench seat beside the gurney.

"Ready?" David calls from the cab of the ambulance. I look at the man and his daughter and wonder, *can I ever be ready?*

"Not yet, give me a few." David turns to glance at me briefly and I shoot him a stare with one eyebrow raised, "Just wait, just wait." I turn my attention to the girl and her father.

"Tell me what's going on," I ask the girl. I do not speak Spanish and my patient, her father, does not speak English. I know the routine better than I should; parents and grandparents, aunts and uncles rely on their children, often too young to read, to translate their pains and injuries to medical providers in emergencies. Children are kept from school to accompany their parents to doctor appointments and are allowed to see their mothers and fathers die because someone needs to translate from Spanish or Hmong (war refugees from mountain regions in Southeast Asia) or Laotian (war refugees from low-lying areas of Southeast Asia) to English and back again. When I was a rookie EMT, we responded to a medical aid for an elderly Hmong woman who spoke no English. Her husband and other adult family members who spoke no English surrounded the woman as she lay in pain, curled up on a couch in a small apartment. We relied on her grandson to translate. But it's difficult to understand a five-year old whose second language is English and the paramedic didn't know how to treat her. How do you treat a severe stomachache? We didn't; we took her to the hospital and let them care for her. She died a few hours later. She had cancer of the stomach, but her grandson didn't know how to say "cancer" and so she was in pain for longer than she should have been. If we had known, we could have requested morphine. We could have made her comfortable. Instead, she died in pain.

This girl speaks English well, though. Her father has been in pain all night and can't stand it anymore. He needs a doctor.

"Why did you call the ambulance? Do you have anyone to drive you to the hospital?" Many people will call an ambulance instead of driving to the hospital themselves, thinking they will be treated faster. But if a patient can walk to the ambulance and gurney, like this man has, the triage nurse will escort him to the waiting room even though we delivered him through the back door.

"We don't have a car," she tells me. No car and I suspect, no friends they can wake up at 3:00 in the morning for a ride to the hospital, twenty miles away.

"If you go to the hospital, how will you get home?"

She shrugs her narrow shoulders. She speaks to her father in Spanish again. I pick up only a few words of the discussion, but enough to know that he doesn't care how they will get home; he is in pain now, not later.

"The doctor will only give you aspirin, nothing else for the pain. Do you have any aspirin at home?"

"No", she says, "We don't have any money for aspirin."

"Ok," I say finally, "I need to see the tooth and call the hospital." I snap on a pair of latex gloves and move toward the man. "Can you ask him to lay back so I can see his tooth?" The girl translates my question. I adjust the gurney into a reclined position and the father rests his head against the rough pillow. His tooth is abscessed beyond repair, the black shell of what it used to be hangs between other teeth that will see the same fate fairly soon. The stench—not morning breath stench but rotting flesh stench—knocks me back onto the bench. I wonder how he has been able to stand the pain until now.

The nurse on duty who answers my call is not happy. "A toothache?" she asks me, not believing what I have said. I called her so she will know I tried to convince the patient not to go to the hospital, because if I bring them a toothache at 3:00 in the morning, they will question everything I do later.

"Yes," I confirm, "a toothache. I've advised the patient that treatment at the hospital will be equivalent to over the counter aspirin. He is adamant in his desire to be transported to the hospital." She makes me wait for her reply.

"Copy Westside, ETA?"

"ETA twenty-five minutes. Do you have any orders for me?" Maybe she'll let me give him a little morphine on the drive, but I don't want to ask her for it directly. If anyone else is listening, I'll be a laughingstock. But the nurse says "no, there are no orders," and I am embarrassed to have asked, although I know my patient needs something for the pain. The nurse has obviously never had a toothache.

Since my patient cannot converse in English and his daughter has fallen asleep on his lap, and there is nothing I can do to treat him. I have time to think on the twenty miles to the hospital; I am surprisingly angry. Not at the patient or his daughter, but at the nurse, for not understanding a toothache and denying the man morphine. And at the way we treat undocumented workers in my town and country. The man refused to give me his name and wouldn't provide any identification, a sure sign that he was undocumented and illegal. How desperate must we make another human before we break them? It is a long twenty miles. The father and I try not to stare at each other for too long but in the tiny ambulance, we catch each other's eyes a few times. I try not to breath through my nose, because the smell of the abscess is overpowering and makes my eyes water.

The nurses glare at me when I escort my patient and his daughter into the emergency department. "Take him to the waiting room," the triage nurse tells me. "Couldn't you do anything to persuade him not to come in?" The mild anger I felt in the ambulance flares and I walk back to my ambulance before I say something I will regret. I am done, I realize. I am done. I can't take any more babies beaten and scalded with hot water. And mothers who extinguish cigarettes on their children and fathers who rape their sons and the people who cover it up. I can't take the woman who goes back to the man who molested her children. I can't take one more boy struck by a car on his way to school and my best friends being shot by their boyfriends. No more drug overdoses, suicides, and near misses. No more. No more nurses who turn their nose up as we walk into the department with a drunk transient. No more. And I can't take any more toothaches in the middle of the night.

The next morning, as I am driving to school, just at the city limits entering Chico maybe two miles from the hospital, I see two figures walking on the side of the road toward me. One is small, dressed in shorts, a light shirt, and flipflops. Her father's polyester coat hangs around her shoulders, draping her like a dress. The other is a slightly built Latino man in his thirties. The man with the toothache and his daughter, who should be home in her warm bed, just waking up to get ready to go to school, are walking the twenty miles back home.

The girl shivers as she climbs into the front seat of my SUV; her father takes a seat in the back. He doesn't say anything when he closes the door, but pulls the seatbelt across his shoulder and tightens it as I shift into gear. I glance at the girl; her pink cheeks warmed in the stream of heat from my dashboard.

"You're not working?" the girl asks.

"Nope, not today," I confirm. I wait while she settles into the seat. "Buckle up," I instruct gently. She pulls the belt tightly and snuggles deeper into the coat. We drive in silence back the way we had come just a few hours earlier. Their little apartment appears even more run-down in the daylight. I wait as the girl's father gets out of the car and scoops his daughter from the front seat. She has fallen asleep somewhere along the way. He looks slightly embarrassed at the situation. I smile, trying to tell him it is okay; she's a kid, she should sleep. I shift into gear as he moves away but then he steps back toward me and I think maybe he has forgotten something. I wait.

"Thank you," he nods slightly. Holding his daughter in his arms, he nudges the car door closed and carries her home.

GRANDMA EVELYN

I spent my entire thirteen years of public education in Orland schools, first at Mill Street Elementary, followed by Fairview, C. K. Price Junior High, and finally, Orland High School. I graduated with 109 of my classmates in June of 1990. I was seventeen years old and eight months pregnant. When I walked across the stage to pick up my diploma in a tent-sized ethereal white graduation gown, my grandmother Evelyn was sitting next to a woman who gasped, "Is that girl *pregnant?*" To which my grandmother reportedly replied, "Yes, and she's *my* granddaughter."

Blood was thicker than water to my grandmother, and I learned from her that you stick by your blood, regardless of the situation. Seven years later, I stood by her hospital bed and watched as she was removed from life support. She had been drying prunes in her enclosed porch earlier in the afternoon when she suffered a massive stroke. She was able to call for help, but by the time she reached the hospital thirty minutes later, blood had seeped through the hemispheres of her brain and had killed any chance at recovery.

Later that evening, we gather at her side, my sisters, my best friend, and mother and I. We talk to her and tell her the stories we remember the most; her heart beats a little faster when we laugh and as I hold her hand, I feel a slight movement, just a tinge. Somewhere, Grandma is still with us. We spend an hour with her before the respiratory therapists come to remove the breathing tube in her throat.

"Its probably best if you wait outside while we do this," the taller respiratory therapist tells my sisters and me. The rest of the family assembles at Grandma's house. We will order buckets of chicken from KFC later, but it will be thrown away in a few days, after the funeral is over, the people who've come to pay their respects have gotten into their cars and told their wives and husbands, "she lived a good life". But I do not think of KFC now.

"I'm gonna stay," I tell the therapist. My sisters and mother look at me, understanding that I will not leave.

"Are you sure?" the tall one asks me, "It could get unpleasant." He holds a syringe and latex gloves in his hands.

"I know," I tell him, "I'm a paramedic." There are privileges to being a paramedic; I get to stay with my grandmother. My left hand tightens around my grandmother's and with my right thumb, I softly stroke the narrow rise between her dark eyebrows. A crease that I have never seen softened runs perfectly straight up and down her forehead; the area around the line is dark from the sun, the line is pale cream.

"I thought you looked familiar," the other therapist says, "where do you work?"

"Westside," I reply.

"That's right," the second therapist confirms. "You can stay if you want, we normally don't like the families to see this. But you know what it is, so," he shrugs his thick shoulders and glances at the tall therapist.

"She wouldn't leave me," I say as I stare at the woman lying on the gurney in the darkened hospital room.

"Ok, it'll be pretty quick," the tall therapist says. I nod

my head and stroke the edge of my grandmother's hair, just above the pale line.

They work quickly to disconnect the mammoth ventilator that breathes in, out, in, out. With one swift motion, the tall therapist uses the syringe to deflate the small plastic bulb that holds the breathing tube in place. With a latexed hand, he pulls the long flexible tube from her throat. They disconnect the cardiac monitor, shut off its blue lines.

I hold her hand and speak to her while she dies, taking in the dark, wrinkled skin of her forehead, the long nails, still dirty and yellowed from digging in the garden earlier in the day, the salt and pepper hair. My family returns to the room and we stand vigil for the fifteen minutes it takes my grandmother's heart to realize her lungs no longer work. I wait in the silence, listening as my sisters cry silently. I feel for the faint pulse of my grandmother's blood as it rushes through her wrist. When my fingers grow numb and her skin begins to cool, finally, I let go.

MARTIN

IT SEEMS FITTING that it would be Martin I worked with my last shift; he had been my first supervisor and my partner more than anyone else. After nearly four years, we knew each other's next move and had developed a synchronized rhythm during calls. We knew each other's strengths and he knew all of my weaknesses. He knew, for me, intubations were a bitch and every once in a while there were patients I cried over. At those times, even if it wasn't his turn to take a patient, he would step up and say, "This one's mine, I need to practice," and I would slip behind him and let him work. He was a big man, well over six feet and 300 pounds. He had been a firefighter and paramedic for fifteen years by the time I came along in the fall of 1993. He knew how to make me laugh and I could make him blush with one glance across the room.

He was married to a schoolteacher when I first met him and had a son just a bit older than my Nicholas. They lived in a little house on the edge of Willows and scraped by like all schoolteachers and paramedics do. There's not a lot of money in either profession, but for people like Martin and his wife, who live to help people, the lack of money doesn't matter much. It's the people, who are important. Once, when I was feeling a little too sure of myself, I shrugged a patient off on Martin and I'm not sure he's ever forgiven me. I had built up a rapport with the patient, talking and flirting with him; he was older and near the end of his life and spent most of his days sitting in a chair in his living room, waiting for his lungs to seize and his heart to stop. He was a "frequent-flyer," we saw him nearly every week as his body was ravaged by the evil that is Lou Gehrig's disease, and most of the time I took care of him. He liked my blue eyes and so I fluttered my lashes for him whenever I could. But on this day, when we went to load him in the ambulance, I told Martin the patient was his. He flashed an angry glare and didn't speak to me for several hours. After building the rapport, I should have stayed with the patient. I let the patient down and to Martin, that was nearly unforgivable. It was a childish error I would never make with another patient.

EASTER SUNDAY—THE LAST DAY

THE LAST SHIFT began at 7:30 a.m. on Easter Sunday, March 31st, 1997. A few days earlier, Martin and I responded to a vehicle rollover out on one of the back roads in the foothills of the Valley, near Black Butte Lake. A group of four men had been fishing all evening and were headed home when their minivan tumbled down an embankment. The men were relatively fine, a few scrapes and bruises. But they didn't speak enough English to tell us they didn't want to go to the hospital, so we decided to transport all of them. Two flew in the helicopter and two rode with me, one on the gurney, the second on a backboard on the bench seat that was normally mine. I spent twenty minutes standing in the back of the ambulance, holding on to the bar that runs the length of the ceiling, trying to treat my patients. I bounced and jostled the entire way. By the time we emerged from the winding, bumpy road, the vertebrae in my lower back had been squeezed beyond repair and my legs were nearly, completely numb. I went home and rested for three days, alternating ice and heat and ibuprofen for the pain. I felt better by Saturday night; it wasn't until the next day, the last shift, when I would began to understand my injury.

On that Easter Sunday, we hoped to get some rest. Maybe, we thought, we'd sneak over to Grandma Evelyn's house to watch the kids hunt for eggs. Grandma's was just across the river and on the way home from the hospital; close enough we could swing in for five or ten minutes. If we could make it that way, we knew there would be a plate of ham and scalloped potatoes waiting for us.

All holidays are different: Christmas mornings in our largely Christian county are quiet except for the occasional kid who falls off his new bike or early morning ham going up in flames. It is only after all the presents have been opened, the last piece of pie has been loaded with whipped topping, and the last guest has left, that someone's grandpa or dad mentions a little pain in his chest or a little difficulty breathing. "Not much," he'll say, "but maybe we should go to the hospital." And someone will call 9-1-1 and we will peel ourselves off the couch and out of our own food-coma, moving slightly slower but still there when called.

Thanksgiving is much the same, with the calls coming just a little later in the evening but no kids falling off of new toys with wheels. July Fourth and Memorial Day are exciting, only because we are responsible for responding to the lake and the river, where overheated mothers and college kids on inner tubes are our most frequent customers. But Easter, with small children hunting brightly colored eggs in the park and families staying close to home, you expect, you hope for, quiet.

We would respond to a total of eleven calls, with eighteen patients between 7:30 a.m. Easter Sunday and 7:30 a.m. the next morning, April 1st. It began with a vehicle collision, and ended with a woman in Hamilton City who had been bleeding into her belly for several days and didn't call us until her breathing became labored and her husband, afraid she would die in his arms, picked up the

Orland biker helped...

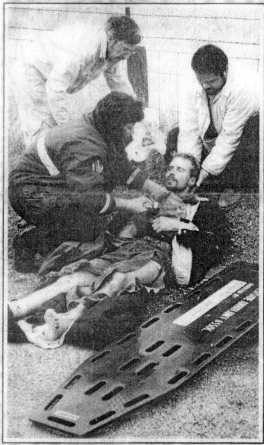

ARTOIS — Paramedic Marianne Paiva, of Orland-based Westside Ambulance, helps calm motorcyclist Michael Mattoon, 33, after an accident on County Road M seven-tenths of a mile north of County Road 30 Monday morning. The 7:53 a.m. accident occurred as Mr. Mattoon was on his way to work. California Highway Patrol Officer Ronald Gleason reports that Mr. Mattoon took a hand off the handlebars to adjust a pants leg when he lost control. He was wearing a helmet. At the scene were volunteer firefighters from Artois and other jurisdictions. Mr. Mattoon was taken by helicopter to Enloe Hospital, Chico. He sustained a broken ankle. (*Valley Mirror* photo by Tim Crews)

Marianne Paiva assisting a patient after a motorcycle collision. (Sacramento Valley Mirror, *Tim Crews*) phone and dialed 911 in the early morning hours of April Fool's Day. By noon, we had already responded to a roll-over accident out on Road 24 and transported a man with chest pain to the emergency department in Chico.

The next call came just before noon; a man in anaphylactic shock waited for us in his small tract home a few blocks from our station. He was the third call on that sunny, perfect Easter Sunday. It came to us as a shortness of breath, that catchall phrase that meant dead babies and drunk men who had been stabbed at what used to be Morrie's Bar out on the highway. It meant grandmothers waiting to die and men impaled on fence posts. When the call came as "shortness of breath," we never knew what we were going to get.

A chrome shiny new motorcycle, a big cruiser that was made for cross-country road trips and whose seat was built for two, perched in the narrow driveway of a clapboard white house. Martin pulled the ambulance close behind the fat tire of the brand-new motorcycle and stopped just short of its tail fin; the ambulance's grill breathed onto the custom leather seat as I opened the passenger door of the ambulance and reached into the patient compartment to hoist a heavy canvas bag into my hand. I lifted my sunglasses and admired the black, still-warm motorcycle as I walked in front of the ambulance, careful not to swing my airway bag too close to the reflective chromed pipes and black paint. As Martin passed the motorcycle, he lifted his trauma bag high overhead and angled his body between the motorcycle and our rig. We ascended the wooden steps of the house to the narrow porch two at a time, our bags of equipment slapping against the sides of our cargo pants as we planted each steel-toed combat boot on the aging steps. It was a well-kept house, at least from the street, but still, as I pinned the boards with my eyes, I worried about the integrity of their nails and crossbars as my feet fell heavily on their faded stain. Martin followed me up the stairs and as I cleared the landing, I wondered how we would carry the patient to the ambulance if he could not walk; our gurney would be a tight fit up the steps, onto the porch, and into the house.

He lay on a small couch in a darkened living room; the pulled blinds and drawn curtains cast the small entryway and room into shades of gray. His gaze moved slightly toward us as we entered, and from somewhere in the house behind him, I heard a woman's voice.

"Yes, they're here now. Yes, yes, I'm sure." She sounded young, at least not aged yet with vocal chords that had been stressed from years of smoking and talking and illness. I imagined she was in her late twenties, pretty in a small town girl way, with auburn hair and dark eyes. I imagined that a decade or more before, she had been the runner-up to the homecoming queen on a cold Friday night during halftime of the varsity football game at the high school just around the corner. If I tried, her name, probably Heather or Melissa or Rachelle, would rise to my memory and I would be able to see her teenaged face before I saw the woman she had become emerge from the kitchen a minute later. She held a cordless phone in her hand as she made the corner into the living room and when she saw Martin and me, immediately breathed, "Oh, thank God." She paused and then spoke into the phone, "no, I won't hang up." She walked toward her husband, whose lips had turned a frightening pale blue in the thirty seconds or so we had been in the house and asked, "How ya' doin'? Are you feeling any better?" and when he slowly closed his eyes and shook his head, she leaned down so their faces nearly touched and with a pale, shaking hand, stroked the soft bangs from his forehead. "The paramedics are here now, everything's gonna be OK." He nodded and turned his head toward the wall, and when she stood, her back was straight and the tears in her eyes were barely visible.

I walk the few steps from the front door to kneel beside a Montgomery Ward couch pushed up tight against a wall, drop my airway bag on the floor, and lean in close to listen to my patient as his chest heaves with each breath. As he inhales, a small, raspy gurgling sound escapes his throat and I imagine the trachea puffy and tender, closing the passage from his nose to his lungs. The pulse at his wrist flutters softly under my fingers and I wonder how much longer his lungs will filter his precious last breaths before his heart will slow to a weak contraction every few seconds and finally stop shortly after, succumbing to the histamine receptors that have been triggered throughout his body. I remember the warm motorcycle in the driveway, notice the discarded leather jacket, gloves, and helmet abandoned by the front door, see the deep red rush of skin at the base of his neck. Even in the small house, I smell the spring flowers that have come to bloom in the past few days and if I tried hard enough, I am sure I can hear the faint buzz of the bees working, flying from flower to flower, depositing their fertile pollen in each open iris, daffodil, and rose they find.

Martin places a large plastic oxygen mask over my patient's mouth and nose, securing it tightly with an elastic band around his head. I rip open the plaid-checked button up cotton shirt and confirm what I suspected; a large welt, the diameter of a golf ball, erupts from my patient's chest, just below the hollow of the neck and less than half an inch from the top button of the light cotton shirt. In the half-light of the room, I find the stinger, still embedded from when the honeybee had aimed at the man's chest and injected its poisonous venom.

I push the man's sleeve up to reveal the soft pale flesh of the crook of his elbow, swab the cool, clammy skin with alcohol, and with the IV Martin prepared for me, plunge a large bore needle deep into the man's vein. His head turns toward me as the point of the needle enters his body, but he fails to open his eyes or make a sound beyond a low mumble at the pain the needle should have caused.

Buried deep in the inner elbow of my patient's left arm, the needle shunts clear fluid from a plastic bag filled with Normal Saline Solution—the equivalent composition of human tears. The saline works to counter the anaphylactic shock caused by the sting of the bee moments before but it will take more than the 1000 mls of fluid in the bag attached to the needle to save this man; his blood pressure is barely audible through the pressure cuff and stethoscope I use to listen for the usually rhythmic thump, thump, thump of the blood rushing through the brachial artery. The artery carries blood from the shoulder to just below the inner elbow, where it splits into an inverted Y and feeds the wrist and hands and fingers oxygenated blood. The brachial is one of the largest arteries in the body, only slightly smaller than the femoral artery in the thigh; if severed above the elbow, the artery could bleed copiously and uncontrollably, causing eventual death if the conditions are right. But as I listen to the faint, erratic shooosh ... shooosh ... shooosh of my patient's pulse through the brachial artery, I know that the anaphylaxis will kill him more rapidly than a severed arm could at this point. The sound of his blood pressure is faint and nearly too slow for me to gauge accurately; I guess that the pressure is somewhere around 70/30, his pulse rate in the 40s. His breathing is shallow and labored; the muscles of his clavicle retract slightly with each breath. His skin, although hot and red on his chest, is cool and clammy on his face. He is in true anaphylactic shock, something I have seen only once before in my career.

Martin pushes a glass vial and needle toward my palm; I

take the clear medication, attach the needle, check the expiration date and the concentration of epinephrine; confirm that the liquid is clear and the vial undamaged. I attach the vial to the syringe, stab the thin needle into the man's thick upper arm and depress the plunger of the syringe, flushing the clear epinephrine deep into his muscle. He winces at the pain of the injection; I take it as a good sign and wait for the sixty seconds it takes for the epinephrine to reach the man's bloodstream. My hand finds his wrist again, finds his radial pulse at the base of the thumb. I close my eyes, drop my chin to my chest, hear Martin shuffle behind me as he uncoils the wires of the cardiac monitor, attaches the leads that will show in what rhythm my patient's heart is dancing.

"What's she doing?" my patient's wife asks Martin.

"Sssshhhhhh," I whisper and wait. Fifteen seconds. Thirty. Forty-five. And there it is, beneath my fingers, the pulse quickens. I count the beat of the pumping blood until it reaches eighty times a minute, grab the stethoscope from around my neck and lean toward the man's chest to listen to the air exchange in his lungs. The wheezing of the lung tissue has lessened slightly but not enough to bring my patient fully awake. I secure the three leads of the cardiac monitor to the man's chest, *white over right, smoke over fire*, and watch as the machine comes to life to show us the secrets that lie in the man's heart. Although he is young, we will have to watch his heart closely because of the medicine we must give him to stop the anaphylactic reaction. I wonder again at the irony of medicine.

***

"I've never been allergic to bees before," my patient tells me as we ride in the back of the ambulance to the hospital twenty minutes later.

"Sometimes you never know," I tell him and shake my

head. "It could be the pollen the bee was carrying that you were allergic to, not the bee itself." He cocks his head and looks at me curiously. I shrug my shoulders. "Keep that to your lips," I tell him and push the nebulizing breathing treatment toward his mouth. The aerated medicine wafts up to his eyes and he blinks uncontrollably.

He pulls the plastic nebulizer from his mouth again. "I thought I was gonna die," he tells me, and I can see the fear in his eyes. "But you see things like this everyday, don't you?" he asks and I know that he's not interested in my career, as much as the possibility of his own mortality. I consider telling him the truth, that no, I don't see death every day, only occasionally. That yes, his own mortality was close at hand a few minutes before. But no, today is not his day to die. Instead, I push the nebulizer toward his mouth again, lean back into the cushioned bench seat of the ambulance, watch cars pass outside the ambulance window.

"I see this all the time," I lie. And when I meet his eyes, he believes me.

The last call came just before 5:00 a.m. After the previous call, Martin sat at the computer completing patient care reports but I had stripped off my boots and had fallen, fully dressed, onto my narrow bed. I didn't bother removing my contact lenses; I assumed that soon enough, another call would come.

We were silent on the ten-minute drive across the valley floor, Code 3, to the woman with shortness of breath in Hamilton City. Martin drove and I rested my head against the cool glass of the ambulance door window and closed my eyes while the early morning darkness swept past us. She would be my patient; the previous call had been Martin's, so I savored every minute of sleep I could tempt sitting up in the seat, sirens wailing every time we encountered another vehicle on the road. Martin would flip the toggle switch up on the panel between us just below the dashboard and then, as we passed the truck or car or van, flip it down.

The house sat in a new cul-de-sac on the street closest to the river; we had evacuated the small town a few months before when the river rose and began to seep through the levee and the sheets of plastic and sand bags the county frantically worked to shore up. The levee held, but we spent three days there, waiting for the water to rush us, calculating how we would escape if the earthen banks gave way. But just after 5:00, before the sun rose on the first day of April, the residents of Hamilton City rested comfortably behind locked doors in the working-class neighborhoods that dominated the sleeping town.

Her husband met us at the door, as most did when their wives were hovering too close to death. Men always want to fix things, and when they can't, they go and find someone who can. Women, on the other hand, wipe sweat from foreheads, fluff pillows, and call out, "Back here! We're back here!" when we arrive. Fluorescent lights filtered from the kitchen into the murky darkness of the small living room. We found her on the couch, where, it seemed, most of our patients had spent the day. She sat on the couch, trying at once to catch her breath while she let her body slump against the thin pillows of the stained fabric of the cushions. Her husband retreated to the middle of the room, somewhere between the living room and the kitchen, and let us work.

Martin kneels in front of the woman, pushes the arm of her cotton nightgown above her elbow, and wraps a small blood pressure cuff around her upper arm. Her husband answers my questions about her medical history: no, she doesn't have any major illnesses; yes, she mentioned a few days ago that her bowel movements looked like tar; no, not vomiting. I watch patiently as the woman labors for each drop of oxygen her small body inhales; her lips, like my bee-sting patient's earlier in the shift, resemble the blue on a summer day and I know, before Martin turns to tell me what her blood pressure is, that we must work fast. Everything I need to know about my patient, even though I know only a few things, is right in front of me. I focus on Martin and the blood pressure cuff, then take a step toward my patient.

"How low is it?" I ask Martin, and he shakes his head as he wraps his stethoscope in his hands.

"Too low, maybe 60 palp," he replies.

"Does she have any veins?" I ask, but I suspect she has been bleeding so long into her belly that her circulatory system has collapsed and we will have a difficult time finding a vein to start an IV.

I kneel next to Martin and we each wrap tourniquets around our patient's upper arms; Martin finds an oxygen mask and fits it roughly over her petite features. She inhales deeply and shrugs into the couch as her body relaxes with the fresh air. I assemble an IV setup and in the pale light of the early morning, search for a vein in my patient's left arm. There is nothing, not a hint of blue or sponginess where a vein should be in her arm and I curse under my breath as Martin examines her right arm.

"Anything?" I ask Martin. His frustration is heavy in the small living room and I feel his answer instead of hear it. My eyes start to tear from exhaustion as I examine the woman's hand for a vein and I realize that I am useless. A small, faint line emerges on the back of my patient's hand but I hesitate to stab it with the needle. "Fuck," I whisper, and Martin glances sideways at the line on my patient's hand. "What if I blow the line?" I ask Martin. "This could be our only shot at a vein." Martin makes a feeble attempt at a vein on the woman's arm, but as soon as he starts to push fluid through the plastic tubing into the needle, a small bubble forms under the skin beside the needle and I know the vein has been compromised.

Hamilton City is the halfway point between ambulance quarters in Orland and Enloe Hospital twenty miles away. Most patients can be transported more easily and quickly from Orland and anywhere in between there and the hospital by ambulance, once the patient is stabilized and loaded into my ambulance. I have made the trip between Orland and Enloe in under twenty minutes, even with traffic. I have driven the eight miles from Enloe to Hamilton City in six minutes. There is no reason, really, to transport a patient from Hamilton City to Enloe any other way than in the back of my ambulance. In fact, it was only when the road was blocked by a fallen tree and the alternate route was over an hour south that I called the helicopter from Enloe and met them in Hamilton City to transport my patient, who was an elderly woman who had just suffered a stroke and for whom every minute without treatment was precious. My stroke patient had recovered nicely because we made the decision to transport her the last eight miles of the trip to the hospital via helicopter.

But my patient with the belly bleed at nearly 6:00 a.m. on April Fool's Day of 1997 didn't have the choice of recovery or not; we could not stabilize her in the field and if she went into cardiac arrest on the eight-mile ride to the hospital, with only me in the back of my ambulance trying futilely to restart her heart without an IV in place, her chances of survival were zero.

Martin stepped to the front entry of the house to use the radio to request the helicopter. The local volunteer fire department responded to set up a landing zone near the house and as the sirens of the fire trucks filled the early morning air, we propped my patient on the gurney, bundled her in several blankets, and waited for the sound of the helicopter as it made the short flight from Enloe to the intersection nearest my patient's home. It seemed like an eternity, waiting for someone else to rescue my patient, and I wondered how much blood seeped its way into my patient's abdomen with every minute that ticked by.

The thunderous crush of the helicopter blades echoed through the silent streets and ricocheted off the houses as the helicopter navigated between the power lines and tall street lamps of the narrow intersection. Martin and I stayed with my patient in her suffocating living room while a firefighter escorted Mike, the flight paramedic from the helicopter, to the house. His thin, lanky frame filled the doorway as he entered the house and without a word, I handed him the IV setup and needle I had prepped. Mike glanced back and forth between my downturned face and Martin's flushed features; he took the needle from my hand and with the slightest effort, placed the needle, threaded the IV to it, and opened the valve that let saline solution run freely into my patient's vein.

"You called us for this?" Mike chastised. He watched Martin, who he had worked with for ten years or more, and when he didn't get a response, Mike stared at me. He waited for an answer.

"I just couldn't see it," I apologized. Mike must have seen the hurt and disappointment in my eyes, or maybe he realized Martin wouldn't have called unless all of his options were spent. Maybe, he saw just how tired we were because he suddenly shifted his stance and relaxed, his shoulders dropping slightly and his arms falling to his sides.

"Do you want to transport? Or should we take her?" Mike asked me.

Martin answered his question when he said, "her pressure is in the sixties; what do you want to do?"

We followed the helicopter as it swept through the early morning light, racing toward the rising sun as it rose over the Sierra Nevada mountain range in the East. I lay my head against the cool glass of the ambulance door window until the next call, the next patient, the next emergency, closed my eyes against the breaking sunrise, and rested while I could.

LOSING JEFF

NOVEMBER 2009

THE NEWS OF the diagnosis came through a friend of a friend. "Did you hear about Jeff?"

"Jeff? Jeff Davis?"

"Yeah, so sad."

Snippets of his deteriorating health filter through our mutual friends over the next two years: He's started losing his strength; he's in a wheelchair now.

A photo of him sitting in his wheelchair on a beach in Hawaii comes across my computer screen in late September. Once strong and tall and a shoo-in for the Majors, the ALS has ravaged his muscles and made his skin glow pink; he has lost his hair. His swollen ankles tell of the failure of his body to function. He gives the camera half a smile and double hang ten gestures with his hands, sunglasses cocked sideways on his face.

October, my husband scolds me: go see him before its too late. But I know I will not.

The news of his death comes through a message posted by one of his children on an Internet social networking site a few hours after he passed. "To anyone who knew my dad:

he died this morning at about 3:00 or so." I post a reply, telling the son of my favorite memory of him and his dad.

Photos flutter across the projection screen throughout the service: There's Jeff, just the year before, taking his first sky dive. There he is in a wheelchair a few months later. There he is with Donna, traveling in an RV the previous summer. An old song from the seventies plays on the stereo system, the wailing voice of Lynyrd Skynyrd singing about a simple man fills the room.

I stand in front of his family and friends, attempt to share my favorite memories of the man I knew, but cannot make the words I want to come. I falter. My voice hitches as I say his name; my heart aches as memory overwhelms my words.

Later, I snuggle with my baby daughter in her bed as I read a book to her before she falls asleep for the night. We turn down the nightlight. I hold her close, let her burrow next to me, both of us buried under a pile of soft blankets. "Mama," she whispers into my hair. I pull her closer, and let my tears dampen the pillow. "Mama," she whispers again, and drifts off to sleep.

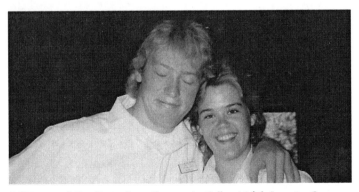

Jeff Davis and Cari Davis, Butte Community College Mobile Intensive Care Paramedic Program, graduation day.

EPILOG

I WAS INJURED in late March of 1997. My knee had been damaged the previous fall, but it was my back that finally went out on permanent strike, leaving me with chronically tingly legs and pain that shoots out to my hips. On good days, I can walk on the treadmill for an hour or more. On bad days, which happen more and more frequently as I get older, standing up straight is impossible. I spent the first Christmas after the injury curled on the couch, watching my son open gifts Santa left the night before. When I tried to stand, the pain ripped through my body and forced me back down. I was twenty-five years old.

I went back to school the following spring semester at California State University, Chico, unsure I would be able to complete the two courses in which I had enrolled. I missed classes, missed quizzes, and more than once, thought about quitting school and returning to my hometown and spending my life working at the local video rental store, watching my old ambulance drive down Walker Street as it rushed to another call. But I happened to enroll in a class that first semester called Sociology of Stress. If anyone knew about stress, I thought, it was me and somewhere in that first semester, sociology clicked. As I read the required text, I

133

felt as if the author (who happened to be a faculty member at Chico) was talking about *me*, and not an obscure theory. I began the class as an English or psychology major (I changed my major at least four times before I graduated) and by the end, was a sociology convert.

Before I finished the requirements for the Bachelor of Arts in 1999, one of my professors said, "You know, if you go to graduate school, they'll let you study paramedics". I signed up immediately and for the last decade or so, I've been studying paramedics. I went back to the ambulance in 2001 to ride along with paramedics and interview them for my Master's thesis and in 2011, I'll return to the field, this time for the dissertation for my doctorate.

Although these stories are from the time I was a paramedic, I found, when I was in the depths of writing them, that I look at them with a sociological perspective. When I was a paramedic, I didn't consciously notice the poverty of Glenn County and the marginalization of minorities, the lack of education or the rampant drug abuse by my patients. Or maybe, because I had grown up there, I didn't want to notice. As a sociologist, I look back and wonder how I could have ever missed it.

It's been over ten years since my last call. I'm married, my son is off in college and we've added a second son and a daughter to our family. I am a sociology instructor at a local college. I'm working on my Ph.D. and spend my days preparing new lectures, doing research about the environment, and grading papers. My students tell me I remind them of their mothers and aunts. They get bored, like all teenagers do when in the presence of uninteresting adults, until I say, "wanna here a story about when I was a paramedic?" and their ears perk up and their eyes come alive, and for a few minutes, I've got them in the palm of my hand. I drive my beat up car, which is pushing nearly

200,000 miles, to the grocery store and back again. I'm fairly normal.

I used to tell people I was a recovering paramedic, kind of like a recovering alcoholic, "Hello, my name is Marianne. I ran my last call ten years ago."

"HELLO Marianne," the other recovering paramedics echo through my dreams.

Sometimes, I wake up in the middle of the night and wonder when the pager will go off. I wait for the red phone to break dreams I have of being back on the ambulance. Sometimes, in my dreams, I feel the arms of my colleagues welcoming me back again and I wonder, each time, when I will be home again.

GLOSSARY OF TERMS

Apneic: Skin tinted bluish due to oxygen deprivation.

Atropine: Medication used to increase heart rate during cardiac arrest; also used to treat pesticide poisoning.

Butterfly needle: A small gauge needle designed with a bandage attached that allows for more secure placement than a traditional needle. Commonly used for pediatric patients.

Chronic Obstructive Pulmonary Disease [COPD]: A collection of illnesses that results in decreased lung function, decreased elasticity on the lung tissue, difficulty breathing, and greater susceptibility to lung infection. Often associated with emphysema, bronchitis, and chronic cough.

Code: The term used to note full cardiac arrest.

Cricothyrotomy: An emergency procedure to secure the trachea by surgically cutting or puncturing the cricothyroid membrane in the front of the neck, and placing a small tube into the trachea when breathing is compromised. Used only as a last resort to secure an airway.

Cardioversion: The procedure of administering low currents of electricity to the cardiac muscle to treat cardiac arrhythmias.

Decompress a collapsed lung: In an emergency medical setting, the process of inserting a large diameter needle through the rib cage, into the lung cavity to re-inflate a collapsed lung.

Epinephrine: A hormone that is used as a medication to treat a variety of illnesses including cardiac arrest, anaphylactic shock, arrhythmias, and low heart rate. The "fight or flight" hormone.

I.V. (Intravenous line): a small catheter inserted into the vein to administer medication and fluid.

Intraosseous infusion (or line): The process of inserting a large diameter needle into marrow cavity of the upper portion of the tibia, just below the knee. In prehospital emergency settings, this procedure is used to administer fluids and medications to infants and young children when intravenous access is unavailable.

Intubatation: The procedure of inserting a large plastic tube into the trachea to assist respiration

Lasix: A diuretic that removes extra fluid from the body. Often used in conjunction with blood pressure control medication to treat hypertension and congestive heart failure.

Nitro (Nitroglycerin): A medication used commonly for treatment of cardiac angina that works to dilate the blood vessels in the heart, lessening pain and decreasing cardiac damage in the event of cardiac arrest.

Running a Code: The medical procedures and medications administered to treat cardiac arrest, which includes cardiopulmonary resuscitation, cardiac defibrillation, and administration of common cardiac arrest medications epinephrine, atropine, and lidocaine.

ABOUT THE AUTHOR

MARIANNE PAIVA EARNED her bachelor of arts and master of arts degrees from California State University, Chico, where she is currently an instructor in the Department of Sociology. She can often be found tending her vegetable garden or walking through one of the many wildlife areas and parks in her neighborhood. She lives in northern California with her husband, three children, two cats, and a dog named Molly.

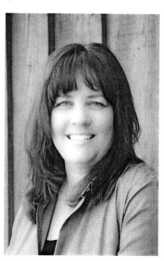

Marianne Paiva

CPSIA information can be obtained at www.ICGtesting.com
Printed in the USA
BVOW081424181212

308401BV00005BA/8/P